THE
SKEPTICAL
PHYSICK

BOOK 2

GAIL AVERY HALVERSON

THE SKEPTICAL PHYSICK

BOOK 2

GAIL AVERY HALVERSON

For Daddy-O

ACKNOWLEDGMENTS

I would like to express my sincere gratitude to Cathi Remlinger-Harding for her boundless enthusiasm and encouragement throughout the writing of both "The Skeptical Physick" and "The Boundary Stone." I am also incredibly grateful to Trish McMahon, Fran Gindera, Anne McMurry and Pam Kleinle, as well as Lisa Genereux, Casey Kane, Katie Roubanis, Paula Mumm, Liza Micheli, Lisa Chizmar, Kelly Risinger, Pippa Goetz, Dawn Byers, Laurie Gregg, MD., Christina Woollgar, and so many, many more. I could not have done this without the love and support of my beautiful mother, Sherry Abbott Avery, my sister, Cindy Hardy, my nephews, Ronnie and Robert Rast, and most of all, the very best husband and son anyone could ever ask for, Rex and Brett Halverson. I love you all.

OF MANY WORLDS IN THIS WORLD

Just like as in a nest of boxes round,
Degrees of sizes in each box are found.
So, in this world, may many others be
Thinner and less, and less still by degree:
Although they are not subject to our sense,
A world may be no bigger than two-pence.
Nature is curious, and such works may shape,
Which our dull senses easily escape:
For creatures, small as atoms, may be there,
If every one a creature's figure bear.
If atoms four, a world can make, then see
What several worlds might in an ear-ring be:
For millions of those atoms may be in
The head of one small, little, single pin.
And if thus small, then ladies may well wear
A world of worlds, as pendants in each ear.

~LADY MARGARET CAVENDISH, 1653

PROLOGUE

"THE WIND MIGHTY HIGH AND DRIVING INTO THE CITY;
AND EVERY THING, AFTER SO LONG A DROUGHT PROVING
COMBUSTIBLE, EVEN THE VERY STONES OF CHURCHES"
~ SAMUEL PEPYS

17 Pudding Lane
Eastcheap, St. Clements Parish
London, England
2 September 1666
12:09am

Thomas Farynor's thick, calloused hands held fast to a wooden handled rake, knocking down the coals of his vast bakehouse hearth with swift, efficient strokes. The sweet, intoxicating fragrance of freshly baked bread hung thick in the timbered cookery of Farynor Bakers, Ltd. Cinders flashed and crackled with every cast, sending glowing bits of ash spiraling aloft before settling back into the embers. Exhaling with unaccustomed exhaustion, Thomas slowly raised himself upright with a deep longing for his feather pallet in the family quarters upstairs. Just past midnight, the stout baker paused but a moment, and yawned, a much satisfied man. It had been an endless, yet vastly lucrative day.

As was his strict custom of industry, after having filled the daily order of two hundred loaves of bread and hard biscuits for the British Navy in their seemingly endless wars with the Dutch, Thomas often worked late into the night to create the sweets coveted by the aristocracy who frequented his shop near the foot of the London Bridge. This day, they had taken a last minute order for ten of his bespoke Banbury pies for the matrimonial ceremony two days hence of young Lady Catherine Abbott to the physick, Simon McKensie. Though time was wanting, he would take great pains with the spiced, dried fruit confections, for with the aristocracy and their extravagant celebrations, it was indeed thinkable that the King himself might favor the intimate gathering with his noble presence. The mere prospect of securing a coveted *Royal Warrant of Appointment* sent an excitable shiver up the cunning baker's spine, for an official warrant made plain in the shopfront window would surely cast prestige, if not a considerable fortune, upon his humble shop—and Thomas Farynor did indeed covet a considerable fortune.

To his utter annoyance, the bride's exacting aunt, Lady Viola Hardwicke, had firstly solicited his oversweet *Pruyme-Taert* wedding pies that had been all the aristocratic rage from the continent. Thomas had groaned to himself when he heard the order, but mindful of the favorable prospects of her trade, managed to keep a civil tongue in his head. Thomas shuddered to think upon the Lady Hardwicke's exhaustive demands during her visit. He thanked heaven above that his twenty-three year old daughter, Hanna, had altered the excitable woman's course, piquing instead her interest in his delicate Banbury pies, for he had put his sizable boot down long before the Lady Hardwicke's entrance into the shop. *Pruyme-Taerts will n'ermore bake in the Farynor ovens! Lord knows the pestilential Dutch—and the loathsome French for that matter—had caused aggravations enough the way they were pouring into the city of late.* Though he feared the loss of her patronage over his dogged refusal to create the spun-sugar confections she desired, Hannah's gentle, soothing ways had becalmed the thorny dowager and after considerable negotiation, the order was at last made. Thomas was especially grateful, for her trade was far too tempting to offend. He sighed once more, weary beyond all measure.

A loud, sharp crack inside the timber-framed bakery startled him from his thoughts. Alarmed, he jerked his head toward the thick oak crossbeams above as a strange and unsettling wind from the east shook the shopfront window. Another gust whistled through the cracks of the bakery's front door, rattling the latch and clattering the wooden shop sign on its rusty hinge outside. A vague sense of unease disquieted the superstitious baker. The beams cracked once more, and then silence fell upon the bakery. He stared up at the rough, hand-planed buttresses for a moment collecting his wits. His devoted old maid, Rose, broke his thoughts.

"'Ere you are, sir," said Rose, setting a wooden tray with a halver of Nottinghamshire Stilton, two soft biscuits and a small earthenware jug of port wine upon the thick pine baker's table with a brisk thunk. "That ought to last ye 'til the mornin' hours, like as not." She sat at a stool and pulled two cups from her apron. She poured them each a dram, and then took a sip, fanning herself with her apron hem.

"My, but 'tis swullockin' 'ot in 'ere, 'tisn't it?" she asked, perspiration beading upon her wrinkled brow.

"Aye, Rosie, it is. It is, indeed."

Rose gave her apron another cooling flick, then tipped her head back and polished off the draught. She set the cup back on the tray and heaved to her feet. "Righty-o then, sir. Till the 'morrow." With a weary heaviness to her steps, she made her way to the narrow stairwell at the rear of the shop. Then, one by one, the old woman climbed the well-worn planks to her tiny sleeping garret two floors above.

"Good 'eve, Rose," he said, casting a watchful eye as her knees creaked on the stairs. *What would I—nae we—have done these many months without her?*

Overhead, the timbers snapped and cracked in the wind once more. Thomas shook off his disquietude and poured another generous quaff of the port. He took up a small pewter knife and sliced a thick wedge of the Stilton. The pungent, earthy scent of the veined blue cheese was a sheer delight to his weary senses. He took a hefty bite. Savoring the sharp, heady flavors of the cheese as it mingled with the fruity port, Thomas leaned against the sturdy table and contemplated his good fortune to be in business still—*nae, even to be alive still.*

Although the devastating plague that had killed nearly 100,000 souls in London at long last seemed on the wane, his beleaguered city was now suffering from yet another crushing blow. The exhausted citizenry were sweltering through an exceptional drought. The bakery, the narrow, twisting lanes of shops, the elegant city mansions and the bursting tenements crowded one atop the other within the massive, stone and wood wall that surrounded the city, were all tinder-dry after the long, parched summer months. *Dear God, how much more are we to bear?* He shook his head and marveled at the resilience of his fellow Londoners. Yawning once more, Thomas polished off the biscuits and the port, and then began to assemble his copper pans, crockery bowls, baking paddles and wicker carry baskets for the morning that would come far sooner than he could gainsay.

Hanna and his young scamp of a son were long asleep in the cozy, timbered nook above the cookery, and Thomas, himself, desperately wished this long day over. At length, he finished his chores. He stretched his aching bones, and then, by the soft, flickering light of his forged-iron lantern, Thomas Farynor himself, finally climbed the narrow, worn steps, tiptoeing through the passageway to his own soft pallet above the storefront window for a precious few hours sleep while the morning's dough rose. Thomas donned his nightshirt and eased his bulk into the cool sheets, running his hands over the crisp cottons that Rose laid smooth each day. He breathed deeply of the thick, sweet scent that permeated his humble dwelling, and thanked God himself for Hanna and Jacky slumbering in the back room. Upstairs in the tiny garret, heavy creaking footfalls followed by a hushed silence signaled that at last Rose, too, had taken to her rope pallet. His eyes fell upon a miniature of his wife on a small table by the bed, her life taken early in the plague's relentless march. He whispered a prayer for her clever soul, and then leaned over and extinguished the candle. The chamber fell into a quiet darkness.

Belowstairs, in the fragrant warmth of Thomas Farynor's bakehouse, one single ember rose on a violent gust of wind that had blown an unlatched window wide to a riot of autumnal stars in a cloudless sky. The ember tumbled sideways, and then rose suddenly, caught in an updraft. The tiny bit of ash sparked. It drifted for a moment suspended on the unseen current, and then tumbled softly earthward. The ember landed, nestling deep into the folds of an errant flour sack that had fallen from the wash basket onto the woodpile. The cinder glowed anew.

CHAPTER ONE

"A WOMAN, A DOG, A WALNUT TREE; THE MORE
YOU BEAT THEM, THE BETTER THEY BE."
~ THE RIGHT REVEREND THOMAS FULLER

St. Bartholomew-The-Less Hospital
Smithfield Parish, London
2 September 1666
12:10am

In the dim light of the dissection chamber, an exhausted Simon McKensie stood and stretched the muscles that burned deep within his sore shoulders. Reaching into the pocket of his tunics, he withdrew a timepiece and held it beneath one in a string of torches suspended from iron hooks upon the rough, plastered walls. Catching the light, he saw to his surprise that it was just past midnight in the now quiet hospital. He turned it over and stared at the engraving on the small golden timepiece, *Gratiam In Appreciation*. Though he treasured this most heartfelt gift of appreciation from the grateful villagers of Wells after his radical medical philosophies had saved so many of them from the ravages of the plague, his heart still ached for the thirteen villagers who had perished. Since his return to London, he had spent many a sleepless night, tortured by the inadequate knowledge, the unknown science that might have saved even those wretched souls. *There is something I am missing*, he thought, gripping the watch in sheer frustration.

He was tired, yet exhilarated by the days research, having worked steadily since sunup on the body of a young soldier who had just that morning expired from yet another resurgence of the Anglo-Dutch wars that had been raging on and off since 1652. *War is but a senseless, execrable waste,* he thought with disgust. Simon took no solace in the knowledge that the corpus of his research for his treatise on plague isolation had grown ten-fold since the hostilities had flared up once again. He stared for a moment at the strong, regular features of the dead soldier, his right leg lost to a blast, and contemplated the deep tub of blood that had collected beneath his grave wounds. *Surely the monumental loss hastened the unfortunate lad's death.*

Simon yawned. He threw his scalpel and brain trepan into a wooden bucket at his feet, splashing cold water onto the freshly swept planks. He looked over to an exhausted Catherine Abbott, who had fallen asleep upon the flat illustration table; her head nestled into the crook of her arm. Glimmering strands of copper hair illuminated by the row of iron lanterns above her table fell across the parchment papers she used to illustrate his findings from the dissection he had that day performed. He smiled at the faint snuffling sounds his betrothed made in her sleep and considered his very good fortune. Catherine shifted slightly, knocking an arm into her drawing instruments. A feathered goose quill fell to the floor. Catherine stirred once again, but did not awaken. Simon stared at the writing instrument for a moment, his brow furrowed in quiet contemplation. He picked it up and held it close under the torchlight, examining it from all sides as though seeing a quill for the very first time. He looked down to the dead soldier, thoughtfully rolling the hollow plume in his fingertips. He ran his fingers up and down the shaft, feeling its variegated texture, at once both rough and smooth. An extraordinary idea began to form. He held it under the glowing torchlight once more and took the measure of its hollow barrel.

"Could such an enterprise er'e be thinkable?" he mused aloud.

At the sound of his voice, Catherine woke with a start. Rising hastily, she gathered her errant strands into the plain gold clips she wore while she sketched. "I fear that I fell asleep, Simon. I...I did not hear you," she confessed, a bit chagrined. She watched a moment as he continued to examine the quill. *Was it his unending curiosity? Or, perhaps it was the determined set to his strong, square jaw that she found so intriguing. Maybe it was the furrowed, quizzical brow above the pale lashes and soft, blue eyes that conveyed the fierce intelligence she admired.* She didn't know, but whatever it was, she was deeply in love.

Engrossed in his thoughts, Simon was unaware of her contemplative musings. "Let us first understand the facts..." His voice trailed off as he stared at the leg of the dead soldier.

"I beg your pardon?" asked Catherine. She hadn't been listening. She quickly gathered her wits and tried to understand his thoughts.

Simon turned to her with his full attention. "Aristotle said that." He held the quill out for her to examine. Catherine took the quill in hand, a curious look upon her face. "Let us first understand the facts..." he repeated. Simon paused a moment, hesitating before he dared reveal yet another of his singular notions for fear she think him an absolute half-wit.

Catherine smiled. "...and then we may seek the cause," she said, completing the quote.

He stared at her in sheer wonderment. *Ne'er in his life had he met anyone who understood him so completely.* "How..." his voice trailed off.

"Master Howell, the Abbey tutor, taught us the philosophers. The writings of Aristotle were a favorite topic of discussion."

Simon shook his head, marveling at his great good luck to have somehow found this extraordinary girl and even more astonishing, that in just two days time, she would become his wife. He drew her into his arms and held her tight, cursing himself once more for being unable to express the depth of his love that at last seemed to settle his turbulent soul. He lay his head upon hers, reveling in the soft fragrance of her hair. He instantly felt tongue tied and clumsy. *He was so very inadequate in expressing his thoughts, in confessing his love for her.* He always had been. She tilted her head up to him and smiled, the tiny creases around her eyes crinkling. She knew. *She knew.*

"What facts do you wish to understand, Simon?" she asked, her voice a whisper in the silent dissectory. She could almost see the thoughts, the hypotheses forming in his mind; such was the dedication, the fervor that seemed to pour from him.

The ideas came in rapid order. "In the study of medicine, you see, Hippocrates taught that illness is caused by an imbalance in the four humours. He believed that an imbalance of one or more of the humours could be cured by the removal of the blood from the body." Simon stared at the soldier's leg, deep in concentration. "And yet, this soldier is dead from far too great a loss of blood." He turned to her, impassioned words tumbling from his mouth. "Perhaps Hippocrates was wrong, Catherine. Imagine the consequences if the common practice of letting blood from the body were the *cause* of illness or death, rather than the healing of it."

Catherine caught her breath. "People should not accept that a theory is true just because a Greek philosopher once said it was," she said.

Simon cocked his head in surprise once more at the depth of her knowledge. "What?"

Catherine laughed. "Sir Frances Bacon. His work on empiricism was also a favorite topic of discussion with Mr. Howell. He was often skeptical of philosophers who offered theory with no proof."

Simon marveled again at her quiet intelligence, then leaned over the dissection table, gripping the wood with an intensity that belayed his outward calm. "I confess that I, too, am skeptical of theory, no matter the source. Theory is but conjecture and conjecture is but mere opinion if it is not based on scientific fact," he said, banging the table with the flat of his hand to underscore the point. "Observable results advance the knowledge of science—observable results proven by actual scientific experiment." He caught himself, pausing in awe at the momentous theory he was about to set forth, then turned to Catherine and dared to speak aloud the idea that was forming in his mind. "What if it were possible to put blood back into the human body when too much has been lost?"

Catherine stopped a moment to consider the extraordinary proposal, tantalized by the science of it.

"I have read that Lower has successfully experimented on a dog," he said, asserting the possibilities.

She was startled. "My apologies, Simon, but, who?"

"The physician, Sir Richard Lower of Oxford University. He has performed a scientific experiment by letting the blood of a spaniel until it was near-dead, and then transferred the blood of a mastiff back into the spaniel so as to render the spaniel back to life."

Catherine absently bit her thumbnail, pondering such an extraordinary experiment. "But, did the mastiff not die? After all, its blood was let in such amount as to equal the spaniel's, was it not?"

"Indeed it did." Simon nodded in admiration at the clarity of her thoughts. "How did you come upon that conclusion?"

Catherine smiled. "As you once said to me in a courtyard in Wells, sir, Euclidean math. A plus B always equals C. Logical thought is not limited to men," she teased. "And neither is algebra and geometry."

"You've studied advanced mathematics?" he asked, incredulous.

"I'm afraid I was limited to needlepoint and elocution lessons by Aunt Viola." A twinkle appeared. "But, each day, during her afternoon rest, I would slip into the library and sit with Charles and Master Howell for philosophy. Mathematics, too, if she slept long enough. I loved algebra and geometry. Opinion and custom do not matter a whit, only the beauty of the equation. Charles received excellent marks," she winked, "but I was even better."

"You are an absolute wonder."

She blushed at the compliment, and then her practical turn of mind began to consider the complexities of the experiment. "How exactly did the physician accomplish the transfer?"

"I confess I do not know, although I have been most curious to learn." Simon thought for a moment. "Father Hardwicke has written a letter on my behalf to Oxford requesting notes on the research and the scientific measures taken to accomplish such an experiment be sent to me, though I believe there has been no reply to date."

"Father Hardwicke would approve of such an act? Would a priest not think upon it as an intervention of God's will?"

"By all measure he has been most generous with his approvals. His inquisitiveness, scientifically speaking, is of equal accord to his great faith. I have often marveled at how he manages to reconcile the two, since he has given me full authority to direct the dissection theater as I see fit, no matter the legalities of the inquiry. I believe he understands such research to be both a necessary scientific inquiry *and* a glorification to God's gifts of curiosity and intelligent thought."

As they considered the extraordinary prospect, a tiny Anglican nun knocked upon the door frame.

"My apologies for the intrusion, sir," said Sister Rosamond, her soothing, gentle voice a marked contrast to her brisk, efficient ways. "The undertaker has arrived."

"Aye."

Simon nodded as two young orderlies entered the chamber carrying a litter. They set it to the side of the dissection table, and then unfurled cotton sheetings enough to enshroud the young soldier. Catherine turned and looked away.

"With apologies, I fear I can never watch this bit," she confessed to Simon. "It breaks my heart to think of his family."

Simon took her into his arms and held her tight. "And that, is precisely why I love you, full of contradiction that you are. You are born to aristocratic lineage, and yet, you crave knowledge and inquiry rather than idle pursuit. You also possess a scholarly strength and intelligence for this laborious discovery of scientific fact, and yet you remain very much the artistic, compassionate woman I fell in love with that day at the coaching inn." He stepped back, his eyes soft with admiration. "Most people could not lay witness to a dissection without abject fear or affliction; even I could not bear it at first. You are a remarkable woman, Lady Catherine."

Catherine blushed once more, then turned her head and yawned. "In truth, I abjectly fear that I long for my bed chamber," she confessed with a smile.

"Then, I shall secure you a coach, my sweet," he said, tapping a finger to the tip of her nose. He looked over her shoulder toward a third orderly and nodded. The orderly disappeared in search of transportation. Catherine laughed and brushed his hand away.

A sudden cacophony of angry shouts from the adjoining Great Hall interrupted the tender moment, the commotion a sharp contrast to the hushed silence of the small dissection theater. Brushing past the men as they began to prepare the body for burial, Catherine and Simon ran into the cavernous, timbered main hall where they saw a furious drunk berating a young woman at the registration desk.

"Ye damnable bitch!" the man shouted, enraged beyond reason. The girl stood quiet, mute to his violent excoriations.

"I ask your name again, sir!" bellowed the bandy-sized registrar of St. Bartholomew's as he stood upon a wooden stool at his massive English oak desk, at once unwavering in his resolve to maintain the strict order he so prized.

The drunk gave him no quarter. "Jaysus, yer a right lackwit," he swore, lashing out at the registrar.

"Sir, I insist!" roared the registrar once more, stepping down from the stool in white-hot fury. He maneuvered his considerable bulk from behind the desk, waving quill and ledger in his outstretched hands. The drunk managed to focus his blurry attentions on the registrar just long enough to kick out at the curiously agile, fat little man who dove back behind his desk to avoid the mud-caked boot coming at him. "Sodding bastard," cursed the registrar, throwing his quill to the floor in irritation.

Outraged howls of protest ringing through the crowded hall created a disorienting pandemonium. From a distant row of rope beds, a crudely carved wooden ladle was flung toward the drunk in sheer irritation. Flying end around end, water droplets splattered over feverishly ill patients. The ladle narrowly missed its mark and landed, racketing across the oaken planks. The drunk held one arm out at an awkward angle. Without warning, he raised his good arm and landed a vicious back-slap across the woman's face, swiftly drawing blood from a split lip. She stood unmoving, her head bowed, absorbing his blows.

"Ye broke me arm, ye brainless twit!" He recoiled from the sight of her. "Aye, God, yer both deaf *and* dumb fer standin' there starin' the way ye do. 'Tis the devil's eyes 'imself, they are, an' no mistake!" Suddenly spooked, he backed away, throwing his good hand out for divine intervention. "Jaysus, the shakin's, the starin's—why, yer cursed, girl," he cried. The man shuddered in fear, then tilted his head in and spat at her feet. "Tha's what ye are… *Cursed!*"

"Sir, I did not see you behind me on the stair," she whispered, bowing her head in shame.

The staggering man lashed out, furious once more. His dirty fingers fell upon the neckline of her striped cotton gown. He gripped the cloth and ripped down hard, exposing her fully to the crowd that had begun to gather. Crude applause and a rowdy chorus of cheers rang out from the back of the hall. Simon was horrified. A sudden memory haunted him.

The vicious beating had left its mark. Stumbling into their drafty shack late from the village pub, his father sat to a plate of stew that his mother, heavy with her fourth child, had left on the course-planked table. Angus McKensie took one bite, and then spit it across the room. "'Tis cold, woman!" he bellowed, slamming the plate to the dirt floor. In a blind rage, Angus had dragged his mother screaming from the bedstead, striking her across the face again and again. The vicious blows left bright red, stinging, welts. In the corner, helpless and hiding under a threadbare blanket, five-year-old Simon watched, his cheeks wet with tears.

Infuriated, Simon was no longer small and far, far from helpless. He charged across the room and gathered the man into his formidable grip. The forcible seizure only served to enrage the drunk.

"Me arm!" he screamed, working furiously to evade the iron grasp that now sent searing bolts of pain shooting through his bones. Wrenching his other arm free, he threw a fist once more toward the silent young woman. Catherine pulled her from the man's reach.

"Enough!" roared Simon, drawing back a powerful fist. He hesitated but a moment; then took lethal aim and landed a crushing blow to the man's bewhiskered jaw.

"Holy shite…" breathed the wide-eyed registrar, as he stood tiptoe on his little stool to get a better view. Though he utterly despised the upstart doctor, the fat little man was nonetheless impressed by the singular display of Simon's youthful, raw power.

The drunk stopped cold as the sensation of blistering pain seemed to work its way through the alcohol-soaked crevices of his brain. He rocked backward and forward on his feet, squinting hard at Simon. *A brief flash of clarity.*

"You!"

A moment later, the sheer agony overwhelmed him. Sagging slowly to his knees, the drunk hit the floor and passed out, cracking his skull upon the scarred planks. Simon stared into the face of the man lying in a heap at his feet. He had seen him somewhere before, yet the association was somehow far from comforting. *Where... Where?* In a sudden burst of recognition, Simon felt his stomach seize. *Flynt Pollard.* A roiling, churning nausea sickened him, for with a single blow, Simon had just rendered unconscious the man that he had paid to exhume freshly buried bodies for his scientific research less than two short years before. Pollard could bring to ruin the reputation he had built with care and hard work, the one man who could bring to ruin *everything* that he had worked so very hard for. To this day, Simon lived in silent fear of being exposed, for exhumations were still a felonious crime, punishable by death, no matter the scientific knowledge gained. *Had Pollard indeed recognized him? Could it ere be thinkable this drunken fool would remember?*

A shuffling sound approaching from behind caught Simon's attention. He glanced back in sudden alarm. Senior physician, Dr. Godfrey Palgrave, passing through the great hall, had laid witness to the forcible takedown. If he thought the late senior physician Alfred Clarke an absolute cretin, the ignorant and superstitious Dr. Palgrave, was far, far worse. An extremist in his religious views and a virulent, pro-exclusion Whig, Palgrave was desperate for power. His deluded lust for Father Hardwicke's position made him all but intolerable to work under, for in his fervent imaginings, Dr. Clarke's miserable death of the plague was but another portent from God signaling his manifest destiny. Palgrave strolled over and set his hands, still stained with dried, rust-colored blood from an earlier letting, upon Simon's broad shoulders.

The fat registrar rubbed his palms together in gleeful anticipation. Not quite tall enough to see over his desk without a stool, the registrar, in his deeply held philosophies, despised anyone who had to duck beneath the low timbered entryway into the great hall. That the striking, muscular physician had straw blond waves that fell to his broad shoulders infuriated the fat little man even more, bald as a parsnip that he was. As a matter of personal conceit, the registrar endeavored greatly to cultivate his own monkish fringe around his balding pate. The graying, wispy strands barely reached his chin. "Aye, yer 'avin' it nae, ye bloodthirsty git!" smirked the registrar, glancing with a shudder toward the autopsy room. In his righteous experience, Simon's dissection theater with its fearfully bloody goings-on was but a sinful abomination to a pious, God-fearing man such as himself.

Dr. Palgrave leaned in close. A lock of greasy hair fell forward, brushing across Simon's cheek. Simon winced as the old man's fetid breath blew hot into his left ear. The physician spoke slowly and with great pleasure to the upstart resident upon which Father Hardwicke had bestowed great praise and privilege.

"Report to Father Hardwicke first thing in the morning, McKensie."

Simon looked down at the drunk, who, groaning in agony, was coming to. He sighed. "Aye."

CHAPTER TWO

Catherine drew the young woman away from the chaos into the deserted dissectory and sat her at the illustration table stool to take closer stock of her injuries. In one of the lanterns above the table, the sputtering flame of a beeswax candle burnt to the quick and broke the silence, startling them both. Reaching for a square of fresh linen, Catherine took a closer look at the young woman and was startled to see that she was but a girl, no more than fifteen or sixteen years of age.

"Can you tell me your name?" asked Catherine, gently daubing at the blood on the girl's lip. A lock of chestnut brown hair fell from her leather tie, obscuring her eyes. Catherine tucked the curl back behind her ear. Unmoving, the girl looked to the floor and said nothing. She clutched the ripped gown tight in her grasp. Catherine could see that although she was shaking from the blows, she held herself with a dignity far beyond her years. A sleeve fell away, revealing a collection of bruises upon the girl's forearm. Catherine drew a quick breath in alarm and asked once again. "Please?" said Catherine, her gentle tone a soothing balm to the injured girl perched on the edge of the stool. The girl glanced at Catherine, as though to take the measure of the woman who seemed to care, then looked to the floor once again.

"MaryPryde," she whispered.

Catherine took note of the torn cloth in the simple, but well constructed gown. The girl sat quiet as Catherine reached for Simon's medical tray. "If you like, I can repair that," said Catherine. The girl hesitated, and then nodded. Catherine took up a needle and stitching thread. She held the needle up to the lantern's amber light and threaded the cotton filament through the narrow eye.

The girl stood, but remained silent. Catherine's heart ached for her. She did not appear to be grievously hurt, but there was a quiet vulnerability that Catherine could not abide. Catherine gathered the torn cloth together and began to work the needle through the fabric. With every stitch, a righteous anger began to swell in her sensibilities for not once in her life had anyone ever taken a hand to her. Catherine was maddened enough to pry further. She folded the girl's sleeve back and ran her fingertips across the angry, red and purple marks with the lightest of touch.

"How did this happen?"

MaryPryde stared down at the discolored welts on her arm, and then touched her fingers to her lip, feeling for the gash that was already beginning to swell. An angry scowl crossed her face, but she held her tongue.

Catherine tried once again. "Has he struck you before?"

The girl looked to the floor, and then lifted her chin and faced Catherine straight on, a momentary spark of defiance flashing in her strange, greenish-gold eyes.

"Aye."

Catherine saw that defiance and pushed further. "Shall I ask the guard to send for the constable?"

"Nae, Miss!" The spark extinguished. "They wouldn'a trouble themselves over the likes of me."

"That's not true, MaryPryde. There must be something they can do."

"For someone like you they would, Miss."

"What do you mean?"

In the silent chamber, MaryPryde hesitated. "I have no money, Miss."

Catherine understood. "I see," she said, nodding softly. Her heart broke at the futility of it all. *One set of laws for those with means, another for those without.*

"Who is that man?" asked Catherine, daring a further inquiry.

The girl looked down again at the floor in abject misery. "Me 'usband," she whispered.

Catherine could not contain the astonishment that overwhelmed her aristocratic manners. "But, you are so young!" she cried. The girl cringed. "Did your parents agree to the union?" asked Catherine, before she could stop herself. She instantly regretted the question for upon the query, MaryPryde seemed to crumble into herself, her very being diminishing before Catherine's eyes.

"I...I have no parents. I have no family." MaryPryde hesitated. "The plague, you see," her voice trailing off.

Unexpected tears filled Catherine's eyes, for she knew all too well that unmerciful pain. Aching still for the loss of her own beloved father to the horrific disease that had devastated the lives of so many, Catherine instinctively reached out to hug the young girl. MaryPryde broke down in her arms.

"I 'ad to, you see, Miss. I... I 'ad no money." Tears streamed down her face. "I was desperate." She looked up to Catherine, eyes wet and ringed red. "So's I took a job." She paused. "At the Ratcliff Alehouse down at the docks."

"Oh!" breathed Catherine, for even she had overheard tales of the disreputable groggery from the sailors who visited her father.

The girl bowed her head, mortified in the extreme. "The position was not what I thought, Miss," she whispered. "I refused 'em."

Catherine understood. "Please do not..."

MaryPryde felt the weight of confession freeing her troubled soul. "I refused 'em, Miss, an' I was sacked." The air hung heavy in contemplation of duties unspoken. "I had nowhere's to go, an' Mr. Pollard offered to take me in." MaryPryde fell silent for a moment. "I imagined it were to cook and clean fer 'im." She stared into the flickering candleflame. "I... I confess that I agreed to the scheme," she whispered. Tears began to fall once more. "Mr. Pollard signed the spousals two days ago an' it were over." She looked to the floor in abject misery.

Catherine did not know how to ask, or even if she should pry, but she felt such a deep compassion for the young girl. She touched the bruises once again. "Did he… did he press himself upon you, MaryPryde?" she dared to ask. MaryPryde turned away, embarrassed.

"Nae. I am yet a maid, Milady," she whispered. "He resolved to it, but I were frightened." Tears streamed down her cheeks as she looked to the discolored welts on her forearms. "I confess I pulled from his grasp and ran down to the lane. But it were dark an' I were lost in that part of the city. So's after a time, I turnt back. By then, he was deep in his cups. He was worse for the drink today." She wiped a tear with a vicious jab. "I…I dinna' know he would strike me." Catherine kneeled and continued to work the needle through the torn fabric, her thoughts a jumble. MaryPryde fell silent.

In the quiet of the dissection theater, Catherine felt an uneasy sea-change. She looked up sharply. A strange and mesmerizing alchemy seemed to have befallen over the girl. Her eyes had turned an eerie and unnatural yellow-gold. Gazing far into the distance, MaryPryde seemed lost in another world. Her fingers began to twitch. Then her entire body began to shake as though caught in a chill. Her teeth began to chatter. For the barest of moments, her eyes rolled upwards so far that only the white orbs were visible. Catherine watched, horrified, helpless as to what to do. Then, as suddenly as it had come upon the girl, it was over. The frightening episode had lasted but moments. Catherine shrank back, afraid to move. Breathing hard, MaryPryde sank to the stool and collected herself.

"How can I help?" whispered Catherine, deeply troubled for the girl. She was wary to touch MaryPryde, and yet could not hold herself back. Catherine knelt down and placed both hands upon the girl's knees. "What can I do?"

"Beggin' yer pardon, ma'am." Sheepish, MaryPryde looked away from Catherine. "'Tis sorry I am that ye had t' see me shakes."

"No apologies necessary, though I am concerned for your well-being. Perhaps we should consult a physick?"

"Nae!" cried MaryPryde, the muscles in her body tensing. "'Tis fine, I am," she insisted. "It only happens when I'm frightened," she said, straightening her spine. "An' I'm not often frightened," she said, in a moment of stubborn pride. Then, in the quiet chamber, the fight went out of the girl. She slumped in resignation. "Me mum called it 'the starin's.' She… she said I weren't to tell a soul." MaryPryde bowed her head, her voice a soft rasp. "She feared people would point and call me a gazingstock. They would say it were th' devil 'imself inside me." She drew back. "Please, Miss, dinna' say anything."

The tinge of desperation in MaryPryde's voice made Catherine's heart ache. She turned her attention back to the needle and vowed to keep her tongue. "Aye, if you like, I'll not say a word."

Eager to change the conversation, MaryPryde reached for a small book on Catherine's table. She looked at the cover, squinting at the title. "A…nat…o…me," she said in a halting voice.

Catherine looked up in surprise. "Are you able to read the whole of the title?"

MaryPryde stared at the writing, then sighed. She set the book back on the drawing table. "Nae Miss. I have no formal schooling, and I canna' write. But I learnt me letters, I did. Me father taught me. He were a bookbinder. I even 'ad a book of me own, but Mr. Pollard threw it in the dustbin when he found it, sayin' it weren't no use of a girl learnin' to read," she frowned.

Catherine took her irritation out on the cloth, plunging the needle back and forth through the fabric with force. "I have heard that sentiment many times before, MaryPryde, but I do not believe it true."

The needle flashing in the torchlight captivated the girl's attentions. "I can sew, Miss. I 'ave me own kit, I do. Aye'n 'tis full of me own supplies. No fabrics though, they was burnt on account'a the plague, a'course. But I 'ave me kit. Me mum said it were a necessity." She looked down at her torn dress. "Sewed me own gown, I did…before he ripped it."

"It's lovely, MaryPryde. You are a beautiful seamstress," said Catherine, examining the tight stitches in the simple but pretty gown.

MaryPryde turned to Catherine her green eyes alight. "I want me own stall in the Exchange, Miss. A dressmaking stall."

"You will be a wonderful dressmaker."

MaryPryde sighed, seeming to reconcile herself to her predicament. "'Tis but a bit of woolgathering, Miss. I s'ppose he's right. 'Tis no use of a girl learnin' th' letters."

Catherine paused a moment, then reached for the book and pointed to the rest of the title. "*Cere'bri. De Anatome Cere'bri.* It is Latin. It means the anatomy of the brain. What the brain looks like inside the head." Catherine held the book toward the girl. "Would you like to keep it?" she asked.

MaryPryde looked tempted. She took the book and leafed through the pages, careful not to bend the stiff, fibrous parchments. A clouded look crossed her brow. She set the book back down on the drawing table once again and this time pushed it away.

"Nae, Miss. He'd never let me have it. An' anyways, I fear I would nae make sense o' the words."

Catherine finished the repair in silence. She tied the thread into a knot and bit it free, then set the needle back onto the medical tray. She turned to MaryPryde and took her by the shoulders. She considered her words carefully. "You do not have to remain with a man who strikes you, MaryPryde. There are…"

A guttural rasp cut short Catherine's words. She felt MaryPryde stiffen in reflexive fear. They turned to see Flynt

Pollard, his wrist bandaged to twice its size, standing in the doorway of the dissection theater. Simon stood behind Flynt, arms crossed, grimly watching over the man's shoulder.

"Girl," grunted Pollard.

MaryPryde backed away, clutching at her gown.

Catherine stepped between the two and faced MaryPryde. "You do not have to go with him," she murmured. MaryPryde hesitated, confused. She looked from Catherine to her husband.

"Now," he growled, his voice threatening.

MaryPryde stood, paralyzed with fear.

"I'm in no mood fer it, you idiotic half-wit!" He turned, banging his wounded arm into Simon. "Damnation!" he shrieked, recoiling in pain.

Simon glowered darkly, and took a threatening a step toward him. MaryPryde remained where she stood, unsure as to which course to take.

In the shadow of Simon's powerful presence, Pollard seemed to find his best manners as he addressed MaryPryde once again. "If y'wouldn't mind?" he smiled, his bearing excessively polite, unwilling as he was to incur Simon's wrath further. Pollard turned away from Simon's watchful gaze. The smile faded as he cocked a threatening eyebrow, then jerked his chin toward the street.

Resigned, MaryPryde gathered her skirts and turned toward the hallway. On an impulse, Catherine took a calling card from her appointment calendar and tucked it into the book; then she took the girl's arm into her own and walked with her. Unseen by Pollard, Catherine slipped the book into MaryPryde's pocket as she departed.

Catherine waited until they walked out of the hospital, then she faced Simon, shaking with anger. "How dare he lay a hand on her? How dare a man lay a hand on any woman? I have certainly heard of such offensive behavior and yet, it is indeed foreign to me in practice. She is but a child—how dare he!" She stopped a moment to calm herself. She glanced toward the doorway. "Perhaps we should notify the constable?"

Simon collected himself, anxious that they abandon the subject of Flynt Pollard. "No!" he said, abruptly.

Catherine looked startled. She turned to her illustration table and began to organize her things.

"I only mean to say that…" Simon's voice trailed off as his thoughts drifted back to the wondrous night they had shared by the fire in Wells, the night he fell completely in love with this extraordinary girl. In those quiet moments, he had at last felt free to confide his crimes of exhumation. To his utter shock, she had not been troubled in the least by his confessions; rather she had been intently curious about the scientific discoveries he had made. *How could she possibly comprehend the peril he still faced, even to this day?*

"My father understood that it is all quite unfair, you know," she said, considering the unfortunate girl's plight. She faced Simon once more, her pale skin luminous in the torchlight. "The way we are born, each to a station," she explained. "Were I, purely by chance, born into her circumstances, would I have learned to read? To write? To study what I pleased?" She picked up the illustration and stared at the precise lines she had laid upon the parchment. "Perhaps this young woman has talents unknown, for how could she possibly bring them to light without the opportunity to try?" Catherine bristled at the injustice. "And, should she now be condemned to a life of misery with that contemptible man, simply because she alone in her family survived?" She looked to Simon, anger flashing in her eyes.

"Aye." Simon turned to Catherine, gathering her into his embrace, much relieved that her thoughts had turned from the constable. "'Tis unfair to be sure."

Behind them in the hall, Dr. Palgrave walked by the open doorway. He stopped short at the sight of the couple, revulsion writ across his face.

"She does not belong here," Palgrave hissed. "Look at her. She is a distraction in the extreme." He placed both hands against the doorjamb, his eyes blazing with anger as he leaned into the room. He stared at the dead man lying on the table, the blood rising in his face. "And her complicity in this...this wickedness, this sin against God, is beyond all reason, McKensie," he shouted, pounding his hands against the doorjamb in frustration. "Beyond all reason!" He narrowed his eyes and glowered at Catherine. "You do not belong here!" He stepped back to collect himself, and then Palgrave turned and shuffled down the hallway.

Humiliated, Catherine pulled from Simon's grasp, her cheeks reddening. She turned to the worktable and began to quickly gather her drawing instruments together. "I must go, Simon," she said, her voice raw with emotion and fatigue. "I... know that I am not welcome here. I am neither nun, nor nurse, and he is not the first man to express the sentiment that I do not belong in the hospital."

Simon set his hands upon hers, gently restraining her. "Catherine, stop."

She pulled her hands from his grasp. "I do not mean to offend Dr. Palgrave, nor do I wish to make things difficult for you," she said, placing the quills into her valise.

"Catherine, please listen. Palgrave has no authority over me nor has he authority over the dissectory. Father Hardwicke has given me absolute imperium over the research conducted in this room." He pulled her quills from the valise and set them back on the drawing table. "More importantly, he has given his full approval to your presence here." He drew her back into his arms. "As have I."

Relenting, Catherine eased into the comforting warmth of his embrace.

"It is my wish that we share equally in what is done here," he said, holding her tight.

An orderly poked his head into the theater. "Your carriage, sir."

"I do not wish to leave you here alone," she said, sleepily laying her head against his chest.

"In but two days time, we shall depart together," he whispered, wondering if she could hear the quickening of his heart the way it did whenever he held her. Simon stepped back and, taking Catherine's arm, escorted her out to the lane. The wind whipped her skirts and tore at the clips in her hair as he handed her up into the coach. He gave the driver two small silver coins. "Bealeton House, St. James, if you please."

The driver nodded, reaching for the leathers. "Get on," he prodded, flicking the reins.

Simon touched two fingers to his lips, and then lifted his hand toward his sleepy bride-to-be as the horse plodded off toward the West End, its hollow, clopping hooves echoing dully down the cobbled lane. Simon lifted his eyes to the midnight sky with nary a cloud in sight. Then, leaning into the ferocious wind gusts that scattered dead leaves in the carriage's wake, Simon turned and walked toward his little thatched cottage on Hawthorne Lane, just outside the massive wooden wall encircling the crowded city.

CHAPTER THREE

Farynor's Bakery, Ltd.
17 Pudding Lane
London, England
2 September 1666
12:11am

In the early morning stillness, caught deep within the folds of the flour sack lying crumpled and forgotten on the bakehouse woodpile, the delicate ember glowed red-hot. The tiny spark dimmed for the barest of moments. Then, the incandescent edge of the smoldering ash caught hold of the coarse linen threads. Gathering strength from the dry winds blowing through the open window, the cinder erupted into a small, ominous flame. The flame burned through the infinitesimal fibers one by one, until at last the whole of the cloth was consumed in fire. The flames began to spread, licking at the fibrous kindling in the woodpile until it, too, was fully ablaze. Merciless in its march, the fire began to scorch its way across the floorboards, reducing the wide-cut planks in its path to blackened char. The blaze climbed the sturdy legs of the vast bakers table, entirely engulfing the pine boards in flames, and then began a relentless crawl toward the rough timbers set deep into the daub walls. A thick, choking cloud of smoke began to drift upward to the timbered ceiling of the baker's shop. It curled around the buttress beams. It seeped through the cracks in the doorway, and swelled up the back stairwell toward the family quarters above. It swirled and tumbled into the front of the shop and filled the back cookery until at last, it billowed out through the open window, a foreboding Angelus rising steadily into the vast, midnight sky over London.

CHAPTER FOUR

Wee Jacky ran through a vast field of summer grain, pulling on the ribbon of a white cotton kite. Though the wheat rose almost to his shoulders, he bounded through the swaying stalks like a newborn puppy chasing the wind. Jacky shouted with glee as the kite soared upwards into a brilliant blue sky, twisting, turning, diving, and then soaring on high once more. Hanna and Thomas laughed, watching the boy as they unpacked a picnic luncheon they had brought in the bakery horsecart. One by one, Hanna lifted the cloth-covered trenchers from a wicker hamper and laid them upon a colorful hand stitched quilt. A joint of cold roast beef. A veal and ham pie. Mutton with smoked oysters. Freshly baked bread. A cabinet pudding. Thomas reached into the mutton pot and lifted an oyster in its shell up to his nose. He inhaled deeply of the thick, wood-smoke and brine scent as he walked to the edge of the field, savoring the sight of his son running gaily in the soft, spring breezes. As he watched the boy, a billowing cloud of smoke off the horizon began to obscure his view. The black, swirling fog spread rapidly across the wheat field, surrounding his son until Jacky completely disappeared from his sight. He turned back to scream a warning to Hanna, but his daughter, too, had faded into the gathering squall. He stood helpless as ephemeral fingers of soot and swirling ash surrounded him. He could not see. The smoke was overpowering, choking his breath; scorching his lungs.

Thomas instantly jerked wide-awake at the smell of smoke pouring through the cracks of the door to his sleeping chamber. *FIRE!* The terrifying word reverberated in his head, for the citizens of London crowded atop one another within the city walls feared no calamity more. Nightclothes tangled around his legs as he leapt from his pallet and fumbled in the dark for the latch. Fingers shaking, Thomas unhooked the iron rod and threw the door open. Thick, choking smoke billowed into his room. An ominous, flickering glow from the bakehouse below threw erratic shadows across his path as he tore through the passageway to the back of the house, banging on the walls to wake the children. Clouds of cinders and ash surging up the stairwell forced a choking retreat back into his room.

"Hanna! Jacky!" he screamed, frantically pounding with both fists upon the plastered wall that separated the two sleeping chambers. He looked to the garret above in horror. "Rose!" He feared her old ears would not hear his shouts. He stood on the bedstead and beat his hands upon the ceiling. "Rose!" he cried, to no avail. For the barest of moments, Thomas stood still atop the straw pallet, helpless as to what to do.

In the bakeshop below, weakened trusses began to fail. Burning timbers snapped and crashed to the ground, the deafening sound reverberating throughout the wooden structure. Shaking walls and heaving floorboards nearly knocked Thomas off the unsteady rope bedstead.

"Father!" Hanna screamed in panic. He could barely hear her over the thunderous roar of the flames. "Father!"

Thomas sprang into action. He grabbed the chair that sat beside his bedstead, and slammed it into the daub again and again, until he knocked a small hole into the plaster. He tore at the hole from his side. Jacky and Hanna ripped at the plaster from their side. Within moments, the opening was large enough for Jacky to crawl through. Hanna kicked again and again at the breach, and then tried to fit through, but the opening was still too small.

"Father!" she screamed once more, stretching her arms through the opening, wildly grasping for him as clouds of smoke began to seep through the cracks in the low, wooden door to her chamber. Within moments, the door exploded in flames, the intense heat melting the iron latch. In sheer terror, Hanna kicked at the plaster once more, this time, widening the gap. She forced her way through to her father's chamber.

Flames burst through the hole behind her. Thomas grabbed the children into his arms and huddled against the wall as the fast-moving flames caught hold of the bed linens, setting the straw pallet afire. *Trapped.*

Thomas raced through the flames to the front window. With no time to work the hinge, he shattered the thin panes with his fist, the glass freely slicing his hands and arms. Ignoring the blood, he knocked the shards away, and then looked down to the lane, quickly taking measure to the distant ground. It was too far a drop. "Hanna!" he screamed over the ferocious roar. The girl ran to his side, shaking in fear. Thomas took her into his arms and hugged her tight. He pointed to the rooftop of the fishmonger's shop next door, and shouted, "Are you able?" She nodded, scared but determined. With the fire burning around them, Thomas helped Hanna crawl through the window. He took hold of her legs and steadied her until she caught her balance. Then Thomas let go. Hanna jumped out and caught the lower edge of the shop's jettied roof. She grasped its corbel braces, hanging tightly to the carved timber. Her palms became wet with the heat and fear. She began to lose her grip. Hanna glanced down to the ground below and panicked. Tears streamed down her face. She looked back to her father.

"I...I'm scared..." she whispered.

"Steady on, Hanna! Reach with your feet!" shouted Thomas.

Hanna took a deep breath to calm her nerves, and then shifted her hands to a more secure hold. She swung out once more, stretching her legs as far as she could. This time, her feet landed securely on the pitch. She threw herself onto the slate tiles and then scrambled to safety atop the roof. Her father exhaled in momentary relief. He could feel the heat searing the skin on the back of his neck. Thomas knelt down to his son. The erratic flames illuminated the boy's soft, innocent features. With his heart in his throat, Thomas took him by the shoulders and stared deep into his eyes.

"Jacky!" whispered Thomas. "'Tis your turn. You must be brave!"

The boy nodded, his eyes wide with fear. With the crackling flames growing closer, Thomas impulsively grabbed his son and held him tight for the barest of moments. Then Thomas lifted him up to the open window. Through the jagged panes, Thomas saw Hanna standing spellbound upon the neighboring rooftop. Her luminous white cottons whipping in the winds stood in sharp, stark contrast to the vast, inky sky. He screamed to her as she stared, mesmerized by the violent gusts that sent torrents of burning ash tumbling and soaring in every direction throughout the narrow lanes. Below, Thomas watched as panic-stricken men and women raced from their homes, screaming for water to douse the flames as they leapt from one structure to the next. In the chaos, several men on horseback wheeled their mounts toward the river wooden buckets in hand. A profound sorrow filled his aching heart. *I fear 'tis futile nae.*

Thomas shouted once more to his daughter standing atop the fishmonger's roof. "Hanna!" His arms were quivering from both fear and the weight of his son. Hanna jerked her attentions back to her father as he held Jacky out the second floor window. She nodded, and lay down on the tiles, anchoring herself as best she could. Thomas kissed his son, and then, in a single moment, Jacky jumped for the truss.

"Hanna!" screamed Jacky. He hung, kicking hard from the beam. He stretched his legs toward the faded red shutters of the fishmonger's shop, trying to gain a foothold. "Help!"

Hanna leaned far over the edge and reached out. Jacky threw a foot out once more toward her. She grabbed his leg just as his fingers slipped from the buttress. Hanna held on tight and pulled him safely up to the roof. Clinging together for a moment, they looked back to the bakery and saw Thomas leaning out from the window, backlit by the ferocious blaze. He was shouting up to the garret.

"Rose!" he shouted. "Rosie!"

"Jump, Father!" Hanna screamed. "I beg you... Jump!" Ignoring her, Thomas continued to shout toward the third floor, but to no avail.

Crawling on his knees, Jacky frantically searched the rooftop around him for something, anything he could find to help. His fingers fell upon a small, broken piece of slate. He grabbed the tile and threw it toward the garret window. It landed short and fell down to the lane with a dull thud. In a panic, Hanna ripped another tile from the roof. She took aim and threw it harder. This time, it hit the mark and shattered the attic's dormer window. Within moments, Rose appeared in her white cotton nightclothes, her hair dangling in two long, gray braids. A fearsome glow illuminated her from behind.

"Jump, Rosie! Jump!" screamed Thomas. In her confusion, Rose could not move. Her old, gnarled hands clung fast to the casement. In desperation, Thomas climbed out the second story window, searching for a handhold in the strapwork. He could see none. He straddled the sill and stretched up to her. "I promise, Rosie—I will help you!" Still, Rose stood, her arms uplifted upon the casement in a silent, almost holy repose. The golden glow grew stronger. A horror-struck crowd began to gather in front of the bakery. Amid the chaos, someone produced a linen sheet. Several men joined together and stretched it to its limit to break the fall of anyone leaping from above. Hanna looked down to the lane glowing in the fire's light below. The bookbinder's shop was now fully engulfed in flames.

"Jump, Father!" screamed Hanna in sheer terror. "Now!"

The heat came at him in ferocious waves. The intensity of the flames burned his skin until at last it became unbearable. Thomas could wait no longer. He looked up to the garret once more, and then reluctantly crawled out of the window. He hung by his fingertips for the barest of moments, and then fell backward, landing in the outstretched sheet. Hanna and Jacky inched their way slowly hand over hand along the rooftops, until at last they came to a window. Breaking the glass, they crawled inside, shouting to wake the inhabitants to the direful calamity, and then raced down the stairway to the lane below.

Huddled close against the unrelenting winds, Thomas, Hanna and Jacky stood with the frantic crowd, watching helplessly as one structure after another along the lane another caught fire.

"Who d'ya's think don'e it?" shouted a man to Thomas.

"Aye! How'd it start?!" shouted another.

Thomas thought fast, knowing the crowd would turn upon him like frenzied wolves 'ere they think he himself had been the cause of their devastating losses. "T'was a man in the night, it was! I seen 'im through me window—'e tossed a fireball into me own shop!" cried Thomas. "T'was… T'was a *Dutchman!*"

The crowd roared. "A Dutchman, indeed!" shouted one man. "Find the bastard!"

"Find the Dutch bastard and hang 'im by the neck!" shouted another, raising his fists.

"Hang 'im by th' neck 'til 'e's dead!" cried more men, still. The mob thundered its approval at the mere thought; crying for the blood of the invading foreigners who they feared were taking revenge for the war.

Up and down the narrow lane, desperate men in nightshirts held fast to sobbing wives and children, watching the ashes of all they held dear scatter into the night skies with the horrific realization that the fire was now far too big to extinguish.

"St. Boltolph's got th' buckets and a ladder!" cried a woman by the side of the lane, watching helplessly as the dry thatch on her home exploded into flames.

"I'll ride fer em," yelled a man, swinging up to his horse. Giving the mare a vicious kick, he raced off towards the Billingsgate church where the fire-fighting equipment was stored.

An ominous crack shot through the lane. Heads jerked toward the bakery as the shop window suddenly exploded, sending splinters of glittering glass refracting in the firelight like faerie dust across the cobblestones. A boy of about fourteen impulsively broke free from the crowd and raced toward the opening. In seconds, he grabbed several loaves of bread from the front table and stuffed them into his cloak. Ducking quickly to avoid a burning piece of wood as it fell to the ground, the boy pulled the hood of his cloak tight over his face and escaped back into the crowd. Incensed, Thomas sprang to life.

"Thief!" shouted Thomas. "Stop that thief!! Stop him!"

His cries of outrage faded as a strange, low rumble emanating from the bakery began to shake the lane. The crowd fell silent, mesmerized by the ungodly sound. Thomas slowly turned back and stared slack-jawed at his bakery, now wholly consumed in towering flames. The rumble turned to an earth-trembling roar. Then, with one single, deafening cannonade, Farynor Baker's, Ltd. exploded high into the night sky. Great showers of sparks soared into the wild, tumultuous winds, flying unheeded toward London Bridge and the Thames beyond. The bakery walls began to weaken, slowly disintegrating into a massive pile of flaming timbers. The roof sagged and groaned, and finally gave way, crashing into burning remains. In horror, he looked up to the garret as the building fell. Rose had vanished into the inferno.

CHAPTER FIVE

Gracechurch Street
Bridge Within, London
2 September 1666
3:47am

A young maid clothed in thick, white cottons and a beruffled nightcap gripped tightly to a turned wooden candlestick. Her calloused hands were trembling, causing the flame to waver. In the dark, foreboding hallway, she stood before a planked bedchamber door and tried to calm her nerves, for she desperately feared disturbing the Lord Mayor of London. Through the thick wood joinery, she could hear nothing but the phlegmy, rafter-rattling snores that were erupting from the old goat. She raised a shaking fist and knocked softly. The mayor groaned. She could hear the finely wrought bedstead creak as he turned about, then a deafening silence. After several anxious moments, she took a deep breath and knocked again. She waited. The bed creaked once more, louder this time.

"Aye," the mayor grunted, after what seemed an eternity. "Enter."

The timid maid lifted the latch, then pushed on the door and stepped into the dark walnut paneled chamber, reeking strongly of stale whiskey and pungent pipe tobacco. She nearly vomited from the stench. In the dark, she tripped on a corner of a needlepoint rug, causing the candle to wobble. She stifled a shriek as hot beeswax dripped onto the back of her hand.

"What the devil?" spluttered the mayor, slowly coming to his wits. He half rose on an elbow and stared in astonishment at the cheek of a maid entering his chamber in the middle of the night.

"My Lord," whispered the maid, nervously peeling the wax from her wrist. "There is a constable downstairs. He wishes to speak with you." The mayor sank back to his pillow.

"Bollocks."

Twenty minutes later, the still intoxicated Lord Mayor Thomas Bloodworth found himself dressed and jouncing in the constable's carriage as they raced toward the London Bridge. Two uniformed tipstaves hung off the back rails, their cloaks billowing full in the driving wind.

Inside the carriage, the constable cleared his throat to break the tension. The mayor ignored him. The silence was unbearable. "'Tis a right tragedy, it is," worried the constable, in an attempt to convey to the highly irritated mayor the scope of the disaster that was currently unfolding in the heart of the walled city. "A right tragedy in the makins'…" He trailed off, for he could see that the mayor was in no mood.

The mayor merely grunted. He pulled on the fabric curtain to block the glow of an oil lantern mounted upon the side of the carriage that illuminated their way through his fashionable district. The light burned his bleary eyes. He laid his head back on the rough leather seat in an attempt to stop the interminable pounding. "I have scant interest in the woes of the unwashed rabble. Even less in taking command of a maidservant's cooking fire," he muttered aloud.

The carriage pulled up to the far end of Pudding Lane and stopped short. The driver stared in horror at the ungodly sight that lay before them and refused to take his rig one inch closer to the inferno that now engulfed both sides of the lane as far as the Thames. Unending clouds of choking smoke billowed skyward. The carriage horses shied and bucked in the deadly shadows, throwing the rig sideways. Panicked men, their faces and clothing blackened with ash crowded around the constabulary carriage, pounding upon the sides, shouting, begging for water and more men to fight the fires. The tipstaves, clinging to the carriage's iron railings, beat the screaming men back as best they could with their wooden truncheons. Their heads bloodied from the ferocious blows, the men refused to back down, clambering instead onto the footboards amid the unrelenting clouds of smoke that obscured the view of the burning buildings.

"Stand back for Lord Mayor Bloodworth," cried one of the tipstaves. "Step back!" The terrified men paid scant attention, desperate as they were for help. Inside the carriage, despite the rocking and pounding that was making him nauseous; the mayor remained where he sat. Moving the fabric window covering aside with a languid flip of the finger, he gazed out at the swirling ash and cinders, at the rooftops ablaze, and at the bakery in flaming ruins. He gazed at the shops and homes afire, then leaned back and closed his eyes in exasperation.

"Shall I give the order to pull down the buildings, My Lord?" asked the constable. For a long moment, the mayor stared out at the fire once more, saying nothing. Without the King's orders for the destruction of private property, he and he alone would be chargeable for all and sundry damages. He thought of his hard-wrought accounts with miserly affection. *God's oath! Such a course would be disastrous.* Unsure of the mayor's hesitations, the constable spoke once more. "My Lord, the men and their longsticks are at the ready. They await your command to pull."

The mayor turned to the constable and fixed him with a long, direct gaze. "No."

The constable was struck dumb. He looked to the raging flames that were spreading from one building to the next before his very eyes. "My Lord, with sincere apologies, the draught, the wind, the dry timbers and thatch, this fire will surely spread. Sir, we must take command of…"

The mayor held his palm up to the constable, interrupting

the man. "Pish," he scoffed. "A woman might piss it out." The constable was shocked to silence by the callous pronouncement. At that, the mayor snapped the curtain closed, and then shouted up to the bench. "Driver, take me home. I wish to return to my bed." In disbelief and shaken to the very core by the Lord Mayor's heartless indifference, the constable stepped from the carriage. The terrified inhabitants of both Pudding Lane and the adjacent Monument Street that had just set to flame instantly surrounded him, crying and begging for help. Ducking to avoid the bits of burning ash cascading in the winds, the furious constable paused, watching the driver slap the reins against the flanks of two skit'tish horses. The carriage pulled away.

∽∾∽

MaryPryde lay wide-awake, staring in a thin slash of moonlight at a wet stain dripping from the ceiling in the cramped attic room Flynt Pollard had let in a dreary Eastcheap boardinghouse. Quiet tears rolled down her cheek, dampening her sleeping bonnet as she thought with such longing of the small but tidy cottage she had shared with her family not one twelvemonth before. She missed the soft touch of her mother's reassuring hands upon her own. She missed the peppery, pungent scent of her father's tobacco. She even missed the daily torment of the teasings and pranks wrought incessantly upon her by her younger brother. She looked up to the small, cracked windowpane, streaked dull from the soot and dross of the filthy East End. It was but incomprehensible to think they were all this day dead. *Though it were indeed a mortal sin against God, dare she think she herself dead, too?* She was abjectly miserable. The deep ache of loneliness and the longing to escape was each day harder to endure. She felt so very alone. MaryPryde wiped away another tear. Lying on the straw pallet next to her, Flynt belched in his sleep and rolled over.

From the street below, an unfamiliar commotion began to seep into her melancholy thoughts. The shouts grew louder.

49

MaryPryde lifted the thin, fraying blanket and stole barefoot from the pallet to look through the garret window. The thin glass did little to dampen the swelling tumult of fearful screams and charging hoof beats that rose upwards from the lane. She drew a sharp breath, stifling an involuntary gasp, for in the pitch-black of night she saw a terrifying orange glow silhouetted just beyond the rooftops of the tenement across the lane. She looked once more to the street below where scores of panicked men were beginning to gather, shouting direful warnings to the inhabitants of Fish Street Hill. MaryPryde began to tremble.

"Fire!" screamed one man, pounding wildly upon the walls of the tenement across the way. "Get out! Fire! FIRE!" He turned and, dodging a multitude of carts and barrows piled high with anything that could be saved, raced to the next building.

On the pallet, Flynt stirred, waking from his alcoholic haze just enough to see MaryPryde silhouetted in a soft light shining through the grimy pane. She seemed to be outlined in a cloud of gold. "What's this, then?" he growled, fumbling over the side of the pallet. He pulled a bottle from beneath the mattress. Lifting it to his lips, he spit the cork to the floor and took a mighty slug.

Though terrified, MaryPryde clenched her fists and forced herself to speak softly, so as to not rile his infuriations further. "'Tis nothing, sir. 'Tis only drunken men fighting in the streets," she murmured, soothingly.

"Christ a'mighty, me arm hurts like God's bollocks," he groaned. He polished off the rum and, tossing the bottle across the room, fell back upon the straw. He closed his eyes in agony. MaryPryde stood at the window. Tipping her forehead against the cold glass, she stared in stark terror at the fire that seemed to be drawing ever closer. Through the pandemonium that roiled through the lanes below, she crossed herself with a desperate prayer that he would fall asleep once more. Long minutes ticked by. She dared not look.

The distinctive, spicy redolence of burning wood filled the cool, night air, seeping freely through the slats and the thin windowpanes of the boardinghouse. She wondered, as she did with every fire that broke out in the congested city, how the familiar scent, at once so warm and comforting, could portend such unspeakable and ruthless destruction. MaryPryde glanced back to the pallet where her husband's breathing had at last become shallow and regular with sleep. She tiptoed across the tiny chamber and quietly changed from her nightclothes into her gown. Retrieving the satchel she had brought with her from the alehouse, MaryPryde quickly packed the few possessions she still had inside. Something hard brushed against her thigh. She put her hand in the pocket of her gown. *T'was the book Lady Catherine had given her.* As she pulled it out, a calling card fell onto the scuffed floorboards. She crossed to the window and examined the card in the soft light shining through the glass. *Bealeton House, St. James Place.*

Without warning, a sudden, massive explosion rocked the boardinghouse to its foundation. She was nearly knocked her off her feet as a fireball ripped through the building across the lane. Showers of sparks and burning ash shot hundreds of feet into the air, whipped every which way by the fierce winds that were roaring through the East End. She steadied herself against the wall to regain her balance, staring in awe at the ferocity of the fire that was now consuming everything in its path. Her heart pounding, MaryPryde began to panic. Men and women poured into the streets clutching their nightclothes and little else, screaming for help to rescue family still trapped inside. The pandemonium was made worse for the carriages racing through the crowds toward the river for water. She looked to Flynt still out cold on the pallet. *A sudden flash of steely resolve.* Flynt moaned in his sleep. *Now. NOW!* MaryPryde took a deep breath, grabbed hold of both her satchel and her treasured sewing bag, and with nary a backward glance, bolted straight through the door.

CHAPTER SIX

"A LEARNED WOMAN IS THOUGHT TO BE A COMET,
THAT BODES MISCHIEF, WHEN EVER IT APPEARS."
~ BATHSUA MAKIN

Bealeton House
St. James Parish, London
2 September 1666
3:47 pm

Catherine sat with Viola at a small writing table in the airy gathering room, leafing through her dissection sketches from the night before with idle fingers. The delicate parchment pages scattered dust particles across the shimmering mahogany grain. Viola averted her eyes to avoid looking at the ghastly images. She leaned over and rapped on the table. Catherine jumped, scattering her papers to the floor.

"Pay attention, Catherine."

"My apologies, Aunt Viola. What did you say?" asked Catherine; leaning down to gather the papers back together. She was still tired and finding it hard to muster an acceptable amount of enthusiasm for the minute details her aunt deemed necessary for a proper wedding celebration. Lifting her own parchment to the light, Viola critically examined the guest list she had worked on for weeks. Though she struggled to see the print, Viola was vain enough not to consider, even for one moment, the leather-framed Nuremburg spectacles sold by street peddlers that would brand her as elderly.

"I said, where shall we place Lord Jermyn?"

"Perhaps he should sit next to Lady Jermyn…"

Ignoring the cheeky impertinence, Viola cleared her throat

and picked up her goose quill. Catherine watched with amusement as, squinting, Viola scratched off one name after the other in an attempt to seat everyone to her satisfaction for the ceremony just two days hence. *Aunt Viola has much changed since the plague confinement in Wells. Indeed, this day, she is a slimmer, calmer, far happier woman.* Heavy lace ruffles on Viola's peacock blue gown fluttered in a strong breeze from the window that had been thrown wide to catch the intoxicating fragrance of the ivory roses in the garden outside. As Catherine watched the flowers bending precipitously in the easterly winds, her thoughts turned to the unfortunate young girl from the night before. *Those who would be kept by men in ignorance might easily be made into slaves.* Her blood began to roil thinking of the brutish treatment handed to the young girl by a man who had deceived her into marriage. *He intended her a slave, indeed.*

"The roses seem to be the only plant in the garden not yet dead from the drought," fretted Viola, interrupting the outrage Catherine was quietly fomenting. Holding her tongue, Catherine glanced outside. Archie Crawdor, estate steward to both Abbottsford Abbey and Bealeton House, stood with her brother, Charles, whose copper curls blazing in the afternoon sunlight were matched in color only to her own. The two were deep in conversation. Catherine smiled as she watched Charles lay an enthusiastic hand upon the back of the steward who, along with several of the Abbey's head staff, had been brought from Stockbridge to London for the wedding. Charles gestured broadly across the expansive terrace, no doubt describing his ideas for increasing the vegetable garden's capacity that he had been researching of late.

At nearly twenty years of age, Charles exuded a raw, newfound strength and confidence hard-gained from his first yearlong navigational apprenticeship to the colonies aboard the supply ship, *HMS Royal London*. Yet, in the broad set of his shoulders, he carried himself with humility and kindness.

He is so like Father. She caught her breath. *Father.* Tired as she was, the still-raw sadness that caught her at unexpected moments overcame her once again at the thought of losing the man they both adored. *T'was a terrible shock upon his return from the colonies for Charles to find Sir Abbott dead of the plague.* Yet, Catherine knew their father would be proud of the way Charles had stepped in to fill the tremendous void his death left behind. *The adversity has by necessity brought about a strength and authority in Charles that may have otherwise taken years to mature. Indeed, the plague hath brought about an unexpected strength and authority in us both.*

Outside, the Lord Mayor of Wells and newly wedded husband to Viola, Cecil Hardwicke, joined the men. He pointed toward the brown, curled leaves that hung listlessly from Viola's prized espaliered pear trees in near-despair, intent upon keeping his wife in good spirits as he was. Viola tried in vain to not look at the ravages the drought had wrought to all but her roses. "Mr. Crawdor will have to ask the gardener to cut the stems at once so that they will be in full flower tonight," she fussed.

"Forgive me, Aunt. What did you say?"

Viola looked intently at the dark circles ringing Catherine's slate gray eyes. "In your fatigue, you've forgotten, I fear, that we have arranged an evening of Master Playford's piano concertos tonight?"

"No, Aunt Viola, I..I had not forgotten." To appease her aunt, Catherine checked the timepiece she wore on a neckbob. "'Tis early still. I promise that I shall rest before supper." She let the timepiece drop and quickly reached for the parchment to study the list, feigning interest. "Who have you placed next to the Earl of Clarendon?"

Viola sniffed at her feeble attempt to distract. "I cannot imagine that you bear the slightest interest."

The two women fell into a quiet moment, broken only by

the sound of a starling's gentle trill from the garden. Viola lifted a reception card, and squinted, pretending to examine the information writ upon it. She spoke softly. "My dear, I must tell you that I do not entirely approve of the time you are spending at the hospital." Viola dared a glance at the detailed anatomy drawings, and then pressed a lace handkerchief softly to her lips in great fear of being unwell. "I might add that this current, revolting subject matter defies all polite custom..."

Catherine lifted her chin in defiance. "Aunt Viola, the knowledge that Simon gathers from his research in the dissecting theater is of the most scientific import," she interrupted, her anger inspired by the thought of MaryPryde's predicament causing a far sharper tone than intended.

Viola raised her eyebrows in surprise, but for once said nothing, for Catherine had been much changed, herself. "Hummph." Viola looked down to her list once more.

Catherine instantly softened. She reached for Viola's hands and took them into her own. She spoke gently. "I know that you would wish a life of wealth and leisure for me. I know also that you are troubled by my marriage to a commoner, but I must tell you that I find Simon's intelligence and scientific curiosity to be of such profound interest and inspiration that I cannot, even for a single moment, bear to think of a life without him at my side. You see, Aunt Viola, I am deeply in love, and..."

"*If* you would allow me to continue, Catherine," said Viola, gently placing a finger to Catherine's lips. "It is true that I do not entirely approve, and yet," she paused, "at almost twenty-two years of age, it *is* entirely your life." Catherine was wide-awake now. "I have not always thought thusly, but I have grown to believe that the words your father spoke before he died were right and true. You must live your life exactly as you wish." Viola smiled at the shock etched upon Catherine's face. "I have indeed learned a good many things since our quarantine in Wells, my dear."

Catherine heaved a sigh of relief and marveled in wonderment at her aunt. The ravages of the plague had leveled all manner of custom in Viola's strict social convictions. *Her marriage to the mayor at the turn of the year has most certainly had a calming effect on her high-strung temperament, as well,* thought Catherine, yielding in her fatigue to a certain impertinence.

As Catherine watched Viola cross another name off her list, the stack of nearly thirty reception cards scattered across the table in a brisk gust of wind. Breathing deeply to calm her irritation, Viola wrinkled her nose at a faint scent of smoke befouling the fresh autumn air. Collecting the cards back to order, Viola cocked an eyebrow and glanced out the window. "Look there," she exclaimed, pointing eastward to a malignant black smudge billowing steadily upwards beyond the elegant mansions of St. James Parish. They both stared in awe at the dense smoke staining the clear azure sky, marveling at the sheer height of the fearsome, swelling plume.

"Why these windows are left open, I'm sure I don't…" Exasperated, Viola caught the eye of a passing maid and fluttered her fingers toward the leaded glass panes. The maid quickly ran to pull the windows shut. "…these winds are positively ruining my hair." Viola looked down and scratched another name off the list. Catherine nearly laughed out loud at the priorities. *Her aunt would never truly change.*

Cedric, the Abbey's ancient butler who had been brought to town for the wedding, intruded upon the moment. Slowly descending the curved marble steps into the sun-filled morning room, he held a silver tray with a card laid carefully upon it. He presented the tray to Viola. "The gentleman awaits in the hall. He wishes to speak to the Lord Mayor."

Viola took the card from the tray and examined it closely. She looked up in surprise. "Mr. Pepys. At this hour?" She glanced out the window. "Fetch the mayor from the garden. Mr. Pepys can join us while he waits."

"Yes, Milady," replied Cedric. As he left, Viola signaled to the young maid standing nearby. "Bring us a tray of tea and biscuits, please," she said, waving to the man standing at the entrance to the gathering room. "Join us, Samuel." He hurried down the steps, a troubling speed to his gait.

"I fear there is no time for a pleasant visit, my dear Viola," he said, reaching for her hand. He bowed, brushing his lips to her fingers with the faintest of touch, and then straightened, impatiently tossing the curls of his dark brown periwig aside. "There lies an impending disaster unfolding to the east of the city. I shall require Cecil's help in securing an appointment with the King in all haste."

The mayor strode with Charles across the gathering room, buttoning the dark gray waistcoat he had opened in the afternoon heat. "What news have you, Samuel?"

Pepys turned to the mayor with the deepest concern. "My dear Cecil, I have just this hour climbed to the tallest point in the Tower of London and can vouchsafe that great swaths of the city center are now consumed in terrible fire. Worse, no one remains to fight it, for every despairing soul endeavors to remove their prized goods, either by flinging them into the river or throwing them onto the barges that lay off shore." Samuel stopped short, stricken momentarily by an incredulous confoundment. "By God's oath, I have ne'er in my life seen such catastrophic destruction on a scale which can barely be imagined."

"Is Bloodworth not there directing all efforts to extinguish the fire?" asked Cecil.

Samuel's curls bounced with anger. "With much dithering and hand-wringing, I'm afraid. The Lord Mayor of London hath indeed a mighty affection and zeal for the King, yet proves himself altogether incapable of managing a kitchen fire, let alone a fire that could well imperil the entirety of the city," he spat.

"Has he not laid witness to the devastation you describe, Mr. Pepys?" asked Catherine, alarmed at the dire tone from a man so customarily genial and light-hearted.

Samuel scoffed. "He has, indeed, Lady Catherine. The constable himself escorted that thickwit down to the East End in the night, yet Bloodworth chose with all haste to return to his bedchamber and slumber whilst the shops and dwellings burnt to the ground. By all accounts, he has not yet returned." He shook his head in disbelief. "I fear he hath no authority to offer…"

"…and will, of course, take none," concluded the mayor. He straightened his cravat and called to the butler standing nearby. "Fetch my walking stick, Cedric." He turned to Samuel. "Have you a carriage?"

"Waiting outside," he nodded, briskly.

"Are *we* in danger?" asked Viola, suddenly much troubled. The mayor placed a comforting hand upon the delicate lace shawl wrapped around her shoulders, then leaned down and kissed the back of her neck.

"Nae, my sweeting. Bealeton House is well-made with stone, brick and marble precisely to resist fire." He pointed to the plumes off to the horizon. "Besides, Samuel vouchsafes that the danger is contained to the east within the city walls, well away from the West End."

"And yet," cautioned Samuel gently, "I fear tonight's programme must needs be cancelled, my dear Viola, as to a man, all will be needed to fight this fire." He was very well aware of the disappointment his words would cause, for Lady Viola Abbott Hardwicke took a very great pleasure in having planned the wedding celebrations down to the last elegant detail. "Perhaps…" he dared venture, "…the wedding should be set by, as well?"

Viola raised her hand in instant protest. "Dare not speak of such a thing, Samuel!" she cried. "I have reluctantly agreed to Catherine's wishes for a small ceremony. I'll not hear of my plans ruined further."

Samuel quickly changed the subject. "And by my honour, I am indeed grateful for the invitation," he allowed in all deference to her prickly temper.

"I shall send a note to Master Playford this hour cancelling tonight's musicale," said Catherine, rising from her chair. "Then, perhaps I might inquire at the hospital?" Jane carried a silver tea service into the room and set the tray upon the writing table.

"Yes, I believe you should indeed, for the needs will surely be great, Catherine," agreed Samuel. "I fear the impending destruction to be absolutely unimaginable."

"Jane, please bring my cloak and handbag."

Viola looked as though she were about to mount a protest, but glancing out the window at the smoke that was growing ever thicker by the minute, the gravity of the situation was well apparent, even to her. She sighed. "Cedric, have Fitch bring the carriage around for Lady Catherine. I shall attend to Master Playford, myself." Catherine kissed the top of her aunt's powdered updo, grateful, in small part, to be relieved of the evening's entertainment. Jane helped Catherine don her cloak, then handed her a small velvet drawstring bag. Catherine looped the bag over her wrist.

"Thank you, Jane," said Catherine as she departed the mansion. "I shall send word as soon as possible."

Samuel looked to Charles standing by the table, taking note of his youth and vigor. "Young man, your strength will be very much required this day. Will you ride with us?"

Anxious to be of service, Charles' eyes lit up with barely concealed excitement. He squared his shoulders and lifted his chin. "I will, indeed, sir." He took a step, and then stopped. He turned to face Viola and Cecil with an unfamiliar authority that none were quite yet accustomed to.

"Mr. Crawdor, I believe that cancelling tonight's programme will free up the staff, will it not?"

"Aye, it will, indeed, Milord."

Charles hesitated but a moment, and then continued,

unconsciously stepping into his father's place. "Please dismiss all available men to help fight the fire."

"Aye, Milord," nodded Archie, approvingly. Charles turned to join the men, then stopped once again with another thought. He turned back.

"And please, if you would, ask Gussie to use all possible Bealeton House provisions to provide food to those fighting the fire. They will soon be weary and hungry."

"Aye, Milord," replied Archie. A broad smile spread wide across his old face as he headed belowstairs, not entirely surprised at the compassion and authority the boy just displayed. "Yer father would be proud," whispered Archie as he passed. Charles turned beet red at the praise.

CHAPTER SEVEN

"I ALWAYS ADMIRED VIRTUE—BUT I COULD NEVER IMITATE IT"
~ KING CHARLES II

Palace of Whitehall
St. James Parish, London
2 September 1666
6:17 pm

A silken coverlet, dypt-dyed in the warm, russet tones of Spanish terra cotta, slid off the top of the bedstead, pooling in a careless heap upon the walnut planks of the spacious chamber's floor. Massive in size, the bed's heavily carved oak posters were topped with a tester hung with crimson velvet hangings. Crowning the tester was a magnificent golden griffin. Giggling, Barbara, Countess of Castlemaine, slid off after the coverlet and landed on the floor with a thud. She impulsively lifted the shimmering fabric to her bare breasts and, peeking above the thick, down-filled mattress, gave a saucy wink to the slender man who lay upon the bed. He exploded in laughter at the bawdy antics of the irresistible temptress. The countess rose slowly from the floor. She stood naked before him in the gilded light of the setting sun, an alabaster goddess as pale and luminous as the carved marble statues of Rome. She was deliciously soft and voluptuous, her body yet plump from giving birth to their second child, a bawling, lusty-voiced lad. The man in the bed could neither keep his thoughts, nor his hands from her; so completely entranced was he by her smooth skin, her sulky, sensuous pout and the merry, teasing wit that kept his sensibilities squarely off kilter.

Barbara crawled back onto the bed and, plucking a golden Mirabelle plum from a lavish basket of fruit, nestled deep into his embrace. She reached up and closed his eyes with her manicured fingertips. Touching the tender, ripe plum to his mouth, she played the fragrant fruit across his lips, tempting him with its velvety down. The heady scent, at once honeyed and thick, evoked memories of languid summer days spent frolicking among the magnificent gardens of St. James Park, days filled with sweet, indolent pleasures of the flesh. The aroma excited him beyond measure. He parted his lips and bit softly through the taut but yielding skin as she traced the curve of his cheek to the cleft in his chin with an idle finger. Gazing into his soft brown eyes, Barbara leaned in close and slowly licked at the juices that ran down his neck.

"Because I will and may not, my will is not my own," she murmured softly. "For lack of will I cannot, the cause whereof I moan…" Her bed-tousled chestnut hair cascaded over the sensuous, heavy-lidded eyes that tempted him endlessly to lust.

"Ahhh, Master Shakespeare…" He gazed at her, as mesmerized now by her unusual, exotic beauty as the day they met. "…thus wisher wants their will, and that they will do crave—but they that will not will, their will the soonest have," he whispered, completing the hypnotic, seductive verse.

She brushed her lips softly across his. He stared into her eyes, the deep, shimmering pools of violet that reflected the fading light through the chamber's towering windowpanes. For the barest of moments, there was a hushed silence.

"And have you, I will!" he cried out, his giddy peals of laughter echoing throughout the opulent suite. He grabbed her by the hand and drew her back into his arms, throwing the velvet hangings closed.

A portly man dressed in a formal scarlet waistcoat with black velvet breeches, stole into the room, then stepped quietly to the curtained bedstead. He waited a moment for the giggling to subside, and then spoke.

"Your Majesty," he intoned, softly.

"Get out," commanded the countess from the depths of the heavily curtained bedstead. She heaved an exasperated sigh.

The man shifted his feet. "Your Majesty," he spoke again, dreading the effect his intrusion would have, for the lady had a famously fiendish temper. The velvet hangings parted. A golden, silk-encased pillow flew out, hitting the man square in the head, knocking his brown periwig to the floor. "Get out!" the countess screeched. She snapped the curtains closed once again.

The man sighed and looked heavenward, begging for patience enough to bear the presence of the woman he so despised. He retrieved his wig and, holding it in the crook of his arm, brushed his own thinning strands back as best he could. "Your Majesty!" he insisted, with all the dignity he had left.

King Charles II poked his head through the rich bedhangings. "Yes, Lord Clarendon?"

The Gentleman of the Bedchamber pretended not to notice his dishabille. "The Lord Mayor Hardwicke of Wells and Mr. Samuel Pepys desire an audience this hour. I fear they bear direful news."

"Damnation!" shouted the petulant countess.

The king sighed. "Show them in."

"Would it not be more seemly to receive them in the Great Hall, Your Majesty?" he ventured, preparing to duck once again. "The Queen awaits an audience with you there as well."

"God's witness, I shall not bear the audience of that dreary girl yet again this day," moaned the countess crawling naked over the covers of the sumptuous four-poster in search of an errant, bejeweled hairclip. "I cannot bear to look once more upon those jagged, yellow teeth," she muttered, the insult scarcely muffled by the thick tapestry bedhangings. She sounded ill at the thought.

The king grinned, his eyes crinkling. "Well, there you have it, Clarendon. She shall not bear it." King Charles II threw the bed hangings wide, laughing at her petulant frown as Barbara sat on the feather mattress, pouting. Her hair hung in loose, brown waves that barely covered her breasts. "Show them in."

Lord Clarendon grimaced and looked away from the countess with utter contempt. The king wrapped the coverlet around his waist and crossed into the anteroom of the massive chamber. He ascended a gilded throne and waited. Within moments, Lord Mayor Cecil Hardwicke, Samuel and Charles were ushered in. At first startled upon the sight of their unclothed monarch, the three men quickly regained their composure and bowed deeply to the King of England.

An exasperated Countess of Castlemaine flounced from the bedstead. Charles' eyes flew wide. He quickly cast his gaze to the intricate, timbered ceiling, trying desperately not to look at the sight of the buxom, unclothed woman gathering her extravagant robes. The mayor stepped in front of the boy, shielding him as best he could. A giddy Samuel could hardly tear his eyes from the spectacular vision of the king's naked mistress.

The countess had worked herself up into a white-hot fit of temper. "Oh, just hand it to me!" she hissed, savagely ripping a dressing gown from the hands of a maid that had been summoned to assist her. The handmaid bowed her head and backed away quietly, well used to the Countess and her thorny ways.

The King watched his paramour as she stormed from the bedchamber and slammed the door behind her, reveling in her fiery temper. The maid discreetly disappeared through a service door and the men were at last left alone. He laughed and turned his attentions to the three incredulous men standing before him. "Gentlemen?" enquired the king. The three men coughed, discreetly clearing their throats.

Samuel took a small step forward, bowing once again. "Your Majesty, there is this day a mighty fire burning in Eastcheap," he ventured, a deeply worried look writ upon his normally jovial countenance. "I fear it to be of such direful consequence that we now beg your immediate concern."

"Has not Bloodworth taken charge?" queried the King, instantly alert.

"He has by some measure been, ahh… ineffectual," offered Cecil, diplomatically.

The king groaned. "Were his attentions not brought to the adversity?"

"He was duly summoned by the constable in the early hours of the morning," said Cecil, with all the diplomatic tact he could muster.

"Yet, at his first opportunity," scoffed Samuel, "the fool retreated to his bedchamber after failing to give the order to pull down the adjacent buildings."

"That ill-considered decision has most assuredly allowed the fire to grow, Your Majesty," said Cecil, his voice now ripe with contempt. "We think it a necessity for you to look upon the calamity yourself."

Troubled, the king considered the predicament set before him. He rose to his feet. Shifting his coverlet tighter, the monarch walked to the window and stood quietly for a moment, gazing down upon the scientific marvel of a telescope that he had installed at the center of the Privy Garden. Standing for hours upon end in the garden, staring through the lens into the night sky was a joy he treasured, for the king was desperate to learn the secrets of the visible world. Fascinated by all manner of science and scientific experiments, the king had even established a laboratory in the castle and conducted experiments himself as a means to promote rational thought and discovery in the populace. It was in service to this rational thought of the populace that he now considered his next course of action. He turned back and looked at young Charles, his red hair glinting in the pale, violet-hued sunset. "You seem to be a young man of strength and wit. Shall we proceed by hoof or by sail?"

Startled, Charles glanced to the mayor. *Should he speak?* The mayor nodded. Charles took a deep breath. "If I may, Your Majesty, Mr. Pepys says the roads are now choked with people escaping the fire. Therefore, I believe the Thames may be the wiser course," he offered, quietly. The mayor and Samuel were both taken by the composure shown by the young lad.

"Then the Thames it shall be." The king turned to his Gentleman of the Bedchamber. "Lord Clarendon, have the men prepare to weigh anchor. We shall depart with all possible speed."

CHAPTER EIGHT

"I AT LAST MET MY LORD MAYOR, LIKE A MAN SPENT,
WITH A HANDKERCHER ABOUT HIS NECK. TO THE KING'S
MESSAGE HE CRIED, LIKE A FAINTING WOMAN, "LORD!
WHAT CAN I DO? I AM SPENT: PEOPLE WILL NOT OBEY
ME. I HAVE BEEN PULLING DOWN HOUSES; BUT THE
FIRE OVERTAKES US FASTER THAN WE CAN DO IT."
~ SAMUEL PEPYS

Westminster
London, England
2 September 1666
7:17 pm

The mansion's jet black, finely appointed carriage worked its way slowly from the West End toward St. Bartholomew's Hospital in Smithfield, a sleepy village that lay just outside the massive 4th century stone rampart encircling the cramped, teeming city of London. Fighting the mass exodus out of the city, the horses sidestepped every few feet and balked at the bridle in fear of the terrified crowds that swarmed against the carriage. Inside the coach, jostling hard over the uneven cobblestones, Catherine clung tight to a polished brass handle and worked to tamp down the dread rising in her chest from an irrational worry that the fire had somehow jumped the thick limestone walls and turned for the West End. Simon's cottage lay ahead in Smithfield. Is he safely away? And what of her friends? What of her publisher, Ambrose Maxwell, who had paid her the highest compliment of her life by publishing her butterfly sketches as a book—what's become of him? And dear Mr. Wilcox, the tailor, who's son, Peregrine, had amused her with his dandified ways before perishing early in the plague. What's become of them—what's become of them all?

As they drew closer to the city, pandemonium raged as fleeing crowds trampled one another in a desperate race to escape the fires. A thick, choking smut of smoke and burnt tar began to drift into the carriage, the overwhelming stench conjuring a sudden memory that was both as ominous as it was detestable. *What was it?* It instantly hit her. *The vinegar.* The unholy fear. The lonely isolation of the plague quarantine. *Her father.* The overwhelming sense of sadness and death hopelessly entwined with the acrid, sour smell of vinegar. *Would she forever despise the scent of smoke as much as she despised the vinegar?*

A movement, a sudden, sharp thud against the carriage startled her from her thoughts. She looked through the window and recoiled from the sight of a soot-covered old man struggling under an enormous pack strapped to his back just inches away from the window. He stared at her for an uncomfortably long moment, and then took a slight step back. He tipped his cap in grand gesture of apology, yet in his glance she saw a subtle accusation. *A judgment. A silent condemnation of the opulent carriage in the midst of profound disaster. A silent condemnation of Her.* He nodded once more, then shifted his baggage and shuffled on, a man alone in a crushing sea of people. She suddenly thought of MaryPryde. Of Gussie. *Of this man.* The sudden rush of guilt weighing heavy. *Each to a station.* She had no determination in her birth, and neither, as she was keenly aware, did they. She put a hand to her reddening cheeks. *She felt his withering contempt, and it stung.* Yet, he did not know her. He did not know how her heart ached for the terrified women racing from the flames, panicked families in tow. For the men straining under heavy loads in a desperate attempt to salvage their entire lives on their backs. For the young children sobbing in fear at the side of the lane, exhausted and unable to walk any farther. *Where will they go, these refugees? What's to become of them?*

Her eyes stung from the fiery ash that blew unheeded through the air, ash that seemed to be drifting toward the palatial homes of the West End and Bealeton House, itself. *Bealeton House.* The thought of the mansion gave her a momentary chill, for Catherine had from the start disliked its cold, marble floorings and the stiff formality of its opulent rooms that were designed to impress. She had never been comfortable with her peerage. *T'was Aunt Viola who had entreated her father endlessly to build the imposing manor house in St. James Parish purely to enhance her own standing among London's elite.* Though Sir Abbott himself cared little for the frivolous habits of the aristocratic set, he had indulged his only sister's whims, for the distraction of building and furnishing the mansion seemed to soften the sharp edges of her flinty demeanor. In truth, he had at last relented to the stone mansion after fire twice burned the family wing of his beloved brick and timbered Abbey in the open, rolling hills of the English countryside. *How she longed for the warmth of the pretty Abbey in the bucolic village of Stockbridge.* The carriage moved on. With dread rising in her throat, she looked through the window toward the massive wall encircling London, now a cloistered deathtrap to the tens of thousands desperately attempting to escape the inferno through its seven narrow, ancient gates. A low moon hanging over the city glowed an evil red through the thick ceiling of smoke.

"Hold tight, Miss," shouted Fitch, as he worked the leathers hard, trying to drive the team through the hoards of panicked Londoners swarming through the lanes, their carts and barrows laden with anything they could carry. Veering to avoid a small boy running across the cobbles, Fitch pulled up sharply on the reins. The two horses bucked and shimmied in violent protest of the sudden yank to the bridle.

"Mr. Fitch!" cried Catherine, as the carriage rocked precipitously from side to side. The handbag on her wrist swung freely against the brass rod she instinctively grabbed hold of.

The coach lurched and creaked, then suddenly lifted high off the ground, suspended for what seemed an eternity upon two side wheels. The carriage wobbled, balancing precariously for a moment. Then, with a violent crack, the rear axle snapped in half under the coach. The back wheel broke apart and fell to the ground in splintered pieces. Time seemed to stand still as the carriage crashed slowly over onto its side. The jagged axel ripped a hole through the bottom of the carriage, leaving a vicious scar scrawled across the cobblestones.

Catherine was thrown from the leather bench to the side of the coach that now lay wrecked upon the ground. She tried to sort her thoughts. *What had just happened?* Disoriented, she gazed around the smoky interior for some measure of balance. The wooden benches were buckled and broken. The window glass had shattered in pieces around her. She took hold of the splintered axel and tried to rise, but to her shock, her strength was gone. Something warm dripped down the side of her face. Bewildered, she wiped it with her glove, and then stared down at the soft gray suede. *Blood.* Her head was pounding.

Fitch had jumped to the ground unhurt, and was frantically working to keep the two costly and very spooked Lincolnshire Blacks from injuring each other, trapped as they were in the riggings. "Your ladyship!" he shouted, struggling to restrain the horses that reared and pawed at the thick, filthy air. He grabbed the yoke and unhitched it from the tangled rigging. Retying the reins to the iron footplate that served as a carriage step, Fitch quickly reached into the feedbag and threw some oats to the ground. The frightened horses began to calm down. They sniffed curiously at the air, and then dropped their heads to the cobblestones nuzzling quietly for the grains. Having settled his mounts for the moment, Fitch struck a flint to the carriage light, then clambered aboard the toppled coach. He threw the door open and gasped at what he saw in the lantern's glow. Catherine lay at the bottom in a bloodied heap.

Fitch leaned into the compartment and stretched his arm down toward her. "Aye, yer Ladyship!" he cried, panicked at the sight of the blood streaming from her head. "I'm beggin' yer forgiveness! T'was the crowd, Miss—they spooked the horses!" Catherine moaned softly. "Take me 'and, Miss." She looked up at him in confusion, her thoughts a muddle. "Take me 'and!" he urged. Fitch stretched farther down into the compartment and, grasping her hand firmly in his, pulled her toward the opening.

Take me hand. Me hand... The words circled round and round in her mind. She could not seem to make sense of any of it. Her knees began to buckle. Her head began to swim. Catherine pulled from his grasp and sank back to the bottom of the carriage.

Alarmed, Fitch jumped to the lane and ran to the back of the coach. He grabbed a rope from a small compartment and, tying one end tightly to the footplate, lashed the other end to the horse's neck yoke. "Hold tight, Milady!" he shouted. He grabbed his leather whip and whipped the horses hard on the flanks, urging them forward. The horses strained against the load. In a panic, Fitch whipped them harder, then harder still.

With one mighty lurch, the horses yanked the carriage upright. Inside, Catherine desperately grabbed for any secure handhold. Finding none, she was thrown violently from the side of the carriage down to the floorboards. The compartment jounced from side to side before finally settling on three wheels. She lay on the boards, stunned, unable to think. "Milady!" Fitch screamed. She flinched as the door was thrown open, and then, as the pain overcame her, the world slowly faded to black.

In the dull haze of the diabolical moon, Fitch clambered inside the coach and pulled Catherine from the carriage. He laid her carefully on the ground. Blood continued to stream from the gash. Fitch grabbed a cloth that was tied to his bench and held it to her head, and then frantically looked around for help as he patted the back of Catherine's hand. At last her eyes fluttered open. Catherine lay still, staring up at him, the edges of her sight blurry. Recognition came slowly.

"What's happened, Mr. Fitch?" She tried to sit up, but the pounding in her head hurt like the very devil himself. She lay back onto the ground. "Please, I…believe I will rest a moment."

"Aye, your Ladyship." Fitch ripped at the silver buttons on his cloak. Throwing it off, he draped the heavy woolen mantle over her shoulders for warmth, and then clambered atop the wrecked carriage to take a better look at the tumult that raged around them. He squinted, lifting his hand to his eyes to block the orange glare from the carriage light. Fitch stared in shock at the sight that had spooked the horses. Stretched out before him as far as the eye could see were untold thousands of terrified Londoners crowding the road in a desperate attempt to flee the city through the single lane opening of the ancient stone arch of Newgate.

"Can ye stand, your Ladyship?" asked Fitch, tearing his eyes from the fearsome sight of it.

She looked up at him, perplexed. "Stand? I…I don't know." She set her hands to the footplate and tried to rise, but the pain in her head made her weak. She sat back down. "I don't believe I am able, Mr. Fitch."

A sudden series of explosions shook the ground beneath them. The carriage rocked violently, nearly knocking Fitch off his feet. He bent down and grabbed hold of the side rack to steady himself as another trio of explosions shook the entire quarter, sending men and women screaming for cover. Catherine looked up to him in confusion and fear. From his view atop the carriage, he could see the source of the explosions. "'Tis the shipping warehouses down at the wharves, Milady. I fear 'tis the oil, tallow, and all t'other combustibles blowing straight up to the heavens."

Fitch climbed down and took stock of the broken axle. He grasped the carriage lantern and took a closer look at Catherine.

Blood dripped down the front of her gown, leaving a ghastly, dark crimson stain upon her fine charcoal-gray woolens. "I shall have to return to Bealeton House for help, your Ladyship, as you are in no condition to ride without a saddle."

In the soft lantern light, Catherine stared at her gloves and gown in disbelief. "Perhaps you should fetch Dr. McKensie from the hospital, instead."

Fitch paused a moment. "St. Bartholomew's? Aye'n I'll bring him right 'round, indeed." He looked to the blood-red moon through the thickening clouds of ash, then down at Catherine sitting so still next to the coach. "I fear the inside of the coach is wrecked. Will ye be all right here, Milady?" he asked, with deep concern.

"I will, Mr. Fitch," she reassured him. *In truth, she felt as though she were about to be sick.*

He quickly scanned the lane now choked with people too frightened to take notice of, or care about, a wrecked carriage. "As you wish, Milady. I shall hurry as fast as e'er I can." He unhitched one of the horses and, taking the leathers in hand, stood on the running board. He swung his leg over the bare back of the horse. Clicking his teeth, Fitch turned north for Smithfield. Catherine leaned back against the carriage to wait. In the deepening shadows of night, the uproar of the crowd slowly faded away. Her eyelids grew heavy. Murky cobwebs clouded her thoughts until she could think no more. *Simon.* Then, in the midst of utter chaos, Catherine lay down to the ground and gave into the overwhelming darkness.

CHAPTER NINE

"WE SAW HOW HORRIDLY THE SKY LOOKS, ALL ON A FIRE IN
THE NIGHT, WAS ENOUGH TO PUT US OUT OF OUR WITS; AND,
INDEED, IT WAS EXTREMELY DREADFUL, FOR IT LOOKS JUST
AS IF IT WAS AT US; AND THE WHOLE OF HEAVEN ON FIRE."
~ SAMUEL PEPYS

River Thames
London, England
3 September 1666
12:07 am

It was a direful sight to behold, indeed. King Charles II, together with his brother, James Stuart, the Duke of York, stood aghast at the bow of the State barge, staring at the colossal inferno burning a massive swath across the city. The king tried his utmost to absorb the sheer size of the fire that was now relentlessly consuming the medieval dwellings of his beloved London. Vast, towering plumes of smoke and brilliant orange flames rose hundreds of feet into the night sky from nearly every quarter. Midnight had turned into day. The warehouses and shipbuilding docks downriver were on fire, as was nearly every building within his sight. In utter disbelief, the king sank to his throne set in the center of the 35-foot shallop, and tried to comprehend the monumental scope of the unfolding disaster.

Creaking, oil-filled lanterns swung erratically on iron hooks, casting eerie shadows upon the murky waters. Churning waves slapped hard against the shallop's wooden plankings. It had taken hours to ply the cumbersome barge upriver. The vicious, easterly winds had slowed the journey to an interminable crawl as the sailors fought hard to keep the shallop on course. The barge's red and gold royal standards snapped above his head. *But by His word the present heavens and earth are being reserved for fire,* thought the king, a sudden memory of childhood scripture flashing through his mind. *'Tis a biblical disaster in the makings, indeed. Neither the city walls nor God himself can contain this conflagration.* In despair, he rose to his feet once more, staring in shock at the enormity of the disaster. *I scarcely believe the destruction that lay ahead for us all.*

In the smoke-filled darkness, six uniformed sailors labored to row the wooden shallop through the turbulent, wind-driven swells, straining to avoid the chattel flung desperately into the river by the terrified citizens. At the rear of the barge, Samuel, Cecil and Charles clung helplessly to the sides of the barge as it tacked hither and thither, banging into all manner of goods clogging the waters. Untold bundles of wood, barrels of ale and wine, even household chairs, chests and tables and nearly anything else that could be hauled down to the banks, bobbed downriver upon the churning tides. An upended harpsichord floating by cleaved a sizeable dent in the side of the boat. Dripping sweat, the men rowed hard in an effort to keep a steady course as the king worked his way toward the entourage in the rear.

"'Tis like the very gates of hell, is it not?" shouted the King over the merciless, howling winds. His gold and deep cobalt blue embroidered cloak flapped wildly around him. Massive flames were now burning uncontrollably throughout the city. A series of explosions from quayside warehouses shot fireballs hundreds of feet into the air, showering the flammable wharves with an unending cascade of sparks and fire. The men ducked to avoid flakes of flaming ash that blew toward them unchecked as the king surveyed the grassy banks that lay between the river and the unfolding apocalypse.

"Hard on steorbord, men! Take us ashore!" commanded the King to the men rowing the barge. The oarsmen pulled hard to the right. Approaching the riverbank in the smoke-filled darkness, the shallop scraped its hull upon the narrow beach as it scudded hollowly onto the rocks. The lead oarsman grabbed hold of a lantern and leapt into the shallow waters. Hauling the barge onto the sandy berm, the sailor lashed its ropes to a nearby tree. As he climbed to the top of the bank, the sailor sank to his knees in terror at the sheer expanse of flames. Without waiting for assistance from his men, the king unceremoniously jumped from the barge and waded through the mud and muck, climbing with James up the grassy bank to take a closer look. King Charles II stared at the inferno in open-mouthed astonishment. *'Tis hell, indeed.* He turned to his brother with an urgency he had ne'er before felt.

"'Tis nothing short of a catastrophe," decried the King, pacing up and down the bank. He shouted to the sailors standing at attention by the shallop. "Horses! We shall require horses!" The King faced James. "Give them coin enough to pay for the mounts," he commanded, his voice low and urgent. James reached into a leather pouch slung across his shoulder and thrust a fistful of silver into the lead oarsman's hands. The rest of the oarsmen scrambled up the bank. Upon the Duke of York's order, the men raced in all directions to commandeer the horses for the King and his entourage. The King paced anew. At length, he stopped and spoke to the men quietly awaiting his orders. "James, I charge you to command all efforts in fighting this disaster. Assemble as many men as may be required to pull down buildings as fast as possible. Spare no house nor merchantry to the west. I will approve any and all measures you deem necessary." He turned to the Lord Mayor, Samuel Pepys and young Charles. "I believe my brother would be grateful for your help in rallying men enough for the demolitions. Are you willing to lend that assistance?"

"Indeed we are, Your Majesty," said Samuel, as the oarsmen returned with the horses. "We are prepared to help in any way possible."

The King watched in despair as his men mounted the horses, then each to a man rode straight into the oncoming cataclysm.

❧

Hooves flying as fast as he dared in the dark, Fitch rode up to St. Bartholomew's and dismounted beneath the whipping shadows cast by a sentinel row of ancient elms blowing wild in the ferocious winds. The driver lashed his horse to the closest tree, and then raced headlong to the hospital entrance. He threw the massive arched door wide and ran to the admittance desk that was thronged with untold scores of injured escaping the fires. Out of breath and panting, Fitch elbowed his way to the front of the chaotic crowd.

"If ye please, sir, I'm t' fetch the doctor."

"Name!" interrupted the registrar, barely looking up.

Fitch removed his driving cap in deference to the brusque little man in charge. "'Tis Fitch, sir, Erasmus Fitch. I'm t' fetch Dr. McKensie," he repeated, working the cap through his fingers. "Oh, an' 'tis a direful plight…"

"'E's busy," barked the exasperated registrar, scratching the driver's name into his ledger with a brown-feathered goose quill.

Fitch leaned over the desk and soundly slapped his hands upon the scarred wood. "I beg of you, sir, 'tis a direful emergency, indeed!"

The toady little registrar looked up sharply, astounded at a blow to his prized registration table. Ignoring the driver's plea, he flicked his pudgy fingers in irritation toward the great hall that was now overflowing with all manner of patients. "The bloody fire's a damnable emergency!"

Fitch turned to look at the teeming crowd of injured, burned and traumatized men, women and children taking refuge in beds, on the floor, in the passageways, even sprawling against the walls of the great hall. They huddled anywhere they could find a bit of space. Some cried out in the most mournful of wailings. Some writhed and moaned in agony from burns to the flesh. Still others sat mute, unable to comprehend the scope of the disaster and profound loss. He turned back.

"But, you see, 'tis her Ladyship, sir," Fitch cried, the desperation in his voice palpable. "Lady Catherine Abbott. She an' the doctor—McKensie's 'is name—why, they're to be married, sir, an' she's been in a carriage accident. 'Tis her 'ead, sir! Oh, an' t'was a fearful lot of blood." He looked sick at the thought. "I'm to collect the doctor, I am!"

"McKensie ain't going nowhere's t'night. None of 'em are," growled the registrar, idly waving his fat fingers toward the arched door. "Get on with ye, nae, or I'll call the guards over an' 'ave ye tossed." Fitch stood, clutching his cap, unsure what to do. The registrar looked over the top of his spectacles and cocked an eyebrow. "Git!" he barked.

Deeply worried for Catherine, Fitch turned and walked toward the doorway, wondering what to do next. He searched the hall for young McKensie, but the physick was nowhere to be found. In his entire life, he had never been at such a loss. *Should he return to Bealeton House for help, or wait for the doctor? Aye'n he'd left her alone on the dark streets—should he return to the mansion for a cart? But traveling back would surely take till the morning hours, what with the fleeing crowds on the streets, so he should wait for the doctor. But, where is he?* He kicked the possibilities around in his simple thoughts. *Which was the right course to take?* He wrung his cap in his calloused hands, desperately weighing both courses. The contemplations made his head hurt. Walking along the wall with the wind whistling through the cracks in the timber joints, he hesitated. He glanced back to the distracted registrar, and then impulsively stopped next to a wheezing old man who sat in a crowded corner, clutching a cloth to his mouth. The man coughed mightily and then glanced upwards, shoving the cloth back into his ragged cloak. Fitch made up his mind. With a polite tip of the cap, wedged his muscular frame down into the scant space left between them.

Fitch was mesmerized by the action swirling around him through the night. The hospital was choked with all manner of people escaping the fires. Every possible set of hands, from the doctors, to the nuns, orderlies and the clerks, had been sent for to attend as best they could to the wounded and dying. Hospital guards had to manage the fisticuffs that broke out by those begging to be seen. The hours slipped by. He no longer knew what time it was, he only knew that he was desperate to find the doctor and return to Lady Catherine. He was about to change his mind and ride for Bealeton House when a tortured, agonized scream startled everyone to silence.

Fitch whipped his head about and saw a tormented woman being carried in on a litter to an empty pallet that sat before a massive stone hearth not far from where he huddled. Rather than touching her to move her to the bed, the orderlies set the litter atop the rope bed. The tiny nun was the closest. Exhausted and overwhelmed, Sister Rosamond gathered her skirts and rushed to the woman, stifling a gasp at the sight of her. It sickened Fitch to the core to see the blistered flesh on the woman's arms and face. Her charred gown had burned the skin on her chest; her skirts were blackened, exposing burned legs underneath. The woman was thrashing on the stretcher in agony. She rolled toward the hearth.

Without warning, a vast tower of logs gave way in a crackling heap. Roaring flames from the fires that warmed the cavernous hall sent a shower of sparks spiraling upward into the chimney. The injured woman screamed once more at the very sight of it, causing a riotous pandemonium at that end of the chamber.

The nun, working to pull the blackened cottons from the woman's body, recoiled in horror at her agonized shrieks. "Dear God! Help," Sister Rosamond cried, casting her eyes about for a pair of empty hands. Every possible doctor, nurse, resident, and even the raw medical students were engaged in the desperate race to treat the injured and dying. Though she had been on duty since the fire began and was exhausted, the nun shouted into the crowded dissection theater for help ministering to the woman's grievous wounds.

"Doctor McKensie! If ye please!" she cried, trying to hold the writhing woman down in a desperate bid to treat her wounds.

Instantly alert at the name, Fitch leapt to his feet and followed her gaze. Simon raced from the overflowing dissectory to help the nun. Fitch cast a furtive glance toward the registrar who was busy barking at a fresh wave of injured crowding his desk, and then ran, ducking, toward Simon as he weaved his way through the beds toward the screaming woman, medical kit in hand.

"Dr. McKensie, sir!" Fitch hissed loudly, waving his cap. Catching up with Simon, the driver matched him step for step as they ran toward the injured woman. "'Tis Fitch from Bealeton House."

Simon stopped short. "Aye, Mr. Fitch! Is there trouble?"

"I'm sorry to tell ye that Lady Catherine's been 'urt!" Fitch looked to the ground overcome with guilt. "The horses spooked. I…I confess I could'na hold 'em to th' bridle at the sight of the crowds escaping the fire, sir." He looked up and faced Simon. "I'm to fetch ye back to Fleet Street."

"How badly is she hurt?" Simon asked, instantly alarmed.

"'Tis her 'ead. Oh, an' there was a right lot of blood. She could'na ride bareback, an' the carriage wheel broke clean off." Fitch clutched Simon's arm. "Would ye come with me, sir?"

"Aye, I will," said a worried Simon. They turned, hastening for the doorway.

"Beggin' yer pardon, sir, there's nae a coach to be 'ad for the fire, an' all. Ye'll 'ave to ride on the back of old Buck wiv' me," Fitch apologized.

The woman in the bed screamed out once again, thrashing in pain.

"Dr. McKensie! Please!" shouted the desperate nun.

Torn between the agonizing thought of Catherine lying

injured in the night and his deep concern for the hundreds of patients crowding the hospital, Simon stopped short. He reluctantly turned back to the burned woman. Watching her for a few moments, Simon took the nun aside. "She'll not live the quarter-hour, if even that," he whispered. Sister Rosamond nodded in agreement, her brows knitted in sorrow.

"Perhaps a poultice of boiled onion mash would relieve her agonies, d'yes think, sir?"

Simon looked skeptical. "Onion mash? Wherever did you hear that?"

"Why 'tis a customary remedy for the burnings, sir. Handed down from the ages, it ''tis," she replied.

"Perhaps this night we shall depend more upon proven science rather than primitive custom, Sister," he said kindly, gesturing to his medical kit. "Hand me the tincture of laudanum, please," he asked.

The nun nodded and quickly reached into the worn leather bag. "Aye'n how much will ye give her, sir?"

Simon knelt down next to the bedside and gently took the woman's blistered hand into his own. "As much as possible."

"Aye, Doctor." Sister Rosamond pulled a small, brown bottle from the leather bag and handed it to Simon. He uncorked it with his teeth, gingerly lifting the moaning woman's head. He spit the cork to the floor. "What is your name, Miss?" he whispered.

In agony, the woman gazed up at Simon, her tortured eyes begging for any measure of relief. "Dorcas," she whispered back. "Will I die?" Simon could not bring himself to answer. Silent tears wet the nun's gorget. He held the bottle to the woman's burned, flaking lips. "Take a sip, Dorcas. It will be of some comfort."

Sister Rosamond leaned over his shoulder. "Take a bit, will ye nae?" she urged gently. Dorcas blinked a silent assent. "Ahh, an' there's a good girl," the nun whispered.

Simon poured a bit of the bitter opium and alcohol mixture into the woman's mouth. Brown liquid dribbled down her cheeks. Dorcas recoiled at the scent of the vile-smelling liquid, and spit it out, but Simon persisted. "Try again," he urged, tipping the bottle once more. The woman grimaced at the foul taste, and then relented, swallowing hard.

"Good girl," the nun whispered, soothingly. "Can ye take a wee drop more?"

The woman closed her eyes and nodded. Simon touched the bottle to her lips. Dorcas swallowed, exhaling deeply. Her eyelids fluttered. Within minutes, her tortured spasms began to subside. Simon lifted her head and gave Dorcas another swallow, watching closely as her body fell limp. He gave her one last sip, softly tracing a finger down her cheek to wipe the spilled liquid. Dorcas opened her eyes and searched his troubled face. Then, with the barest hint of a smile, she closed them once more and slowly drifted away on an ethereal cloud of opium extract. After several minutes, her breathing ebbed, and then finally, mercifully, Dorcas ceased breathing altogether. In the quiet moment that followed, Sister Rosamond crossed herself and whispered a soft prayer. Behind her, Fitch sorrowfully removed his cap and looked to the ground in silent reverence. Simon took hold of Dorcas' hand and, holding it gently, contemplated the extent of her grievous injuries. *How much pain could the human body endure?*

Though he tried to fight it, in his exhaustion, Simon was moved to tears. He sank to the edge of the stretcher for a moment and set his head in his hands, trying desperately to shut out the ear splitting, head pounding cries of the wounded. The great hall was hot and fetid from the crush of people pressed into every corner of the hospital. He looked down to see his tunics now soaked from the sweat, blood and filth from the interminable stream of injured. The thick stench of charred flesh and blood seared into his senses. Across the hall, yet another horribly burned man cried out in agony. *There is no end to this incomprehensible tragedy.*

Wiping his eyes, Simon pulled the timepiece from his pocket.

He was astounded to see that it had been nearly twenty-six hours since he had been summoned back to the hospital from his cottage down the lane. He had collapsed fully clothed upon his bed after the long day in the dissectory. It had seemed but a blink when an incessant pounding on the cottage door awakened him from the sleep of the dead. *T'was a mere trickle at first, but as the desperate hours passed, the injured had descended upon the hospital in near biblical proportions.* There was nary an inch of space left in the entire hospital to treat the fire victims. He, himself, was not sure how much longer he could manage. Simon set Dorcas' hands carefully upon her chest and covered her fully with the rough linen sheet. Resigned, he summoned the nearby orderlies, and then reluctantly arose, searching the hall for Father Hardwicke. *He would have to administer the last rites once more.*

Sister Rosamond placed a comforting hand upon his shoulder. "Ye've had a long two days, sir. Ye ought to go home and take a bit of a snudge. Ye'll be needed later, like as not."

"I'll just find Father Hardwicke," Simon began, unable to take his eyes from the linen covered body.

The nun held up her hand to silence him. "Aye'n I'll speak to Father Hardwicke, me'self," she said, with a sharp waggle of her finger, "an' tell him I bade you to home for a rest." She looked askance to Fitch staring uneasily over the dead woman and raised an eyebrow. "Get on with ye, Doctor." Fitch jumped back, clearing his throat in embarrassment.

Simon reluctantly wiped his eyes, ringed dark with fatigue. "Aye, I will, Sister." He furrowed his bow. "You have been on duty as long as I have. You must rest, yourself."

"We have our chambers upstairs—I will indeed rest. You have my word, Doctor McKensie."

At that, Simon took hold of his medical kit, then took a deep breath and turned to face Fitch, nodding. "Let us depart."

CHAPTER TEN

St. Andrew, Holborn Parish
London, England
3 September 1666
5:47am

A firm hand upon her shoulder gently shook her awake. "Catherine!" The urgent voice intruded rudely into the dream-like, Elysian depths of her slumber. She was so very tired. *Let me sleep.* "Catherine, wake up!" *Please, let me sleep.* Another shake, this time harder. "Wake up!" The clouds in her head began to part. "Catherine!" The voice, loud and forceful, pierced deep into her consciousness. Catherine lay on her back and slowly opened her eyes, trying to fathom where she could possibly be.

The sky above glowed a strange orange. *Curious.* Frantic, teeming crowds of people raced by, neither looking at nor caring about the upended carriage or it's injured occupant. She looked at the riggings that lay tangled on the ground. The horse was gone. *How long have I been here?* She glanced at her wrist. Her handbag was missing. *Is it day or is it night?* She touched her fingers to her neck. Her timepiece had been stolen, as were the small, pearl earbobs given to her by her father. Her shoes were missing. Even the gold clips in her hair had been nicked. *What's happened?* A piercing stab of pain lodged over her left temple. Choking smoke seized her lungs. She began to cough. Her eyes stung as her sight began to focus through the smoky haze. Simon knelt above her, backlit by the odd, yellow sky, his eyes knitted in deep concern. He held the carriage lantern up. The bright glow of the oil lamp pierced her eyes. "Catherine!" She struggled to rise, trying to shake the cobwebs from her mind. She looked over to the wrecked carriage, and then up to Simon. *Simon.* Fitch stood nearby, anxiously crushing his cap between his fingers. *She was terribly confused.*

"What's happened?" she said, aloud. Her voice sounded odd. *Nothing seemed familiar.*

"Ye've had a blow to the 'ead, Miss," blurted Fitch, much troubled by her injuries. "The horses spooked, 'an I lost control of the carriage. I canna' apologize enough t' ye, yer Ladyship." He looked as though he were about to cry.

Simon knelt down and took hold of her bare feet, testing first her right leg and then the left for signs of breakage. "Catherine, how do you feel?"

Her manners were instinctive. "I…I am fine." She sat up slowly, the clouds beginning to clear.

"Nae, Catherine. Can you tell me how you *feel?*" he asked again.

She stared at him for a moment, and then realized what he was asking. *Scientifically.* He was asking for a scientific answer. She sat up and slowly took stock, moving her arms and legs, her hands and feet. "I have no broken bones. My head hurts. I…I can't seem to collect my thoughts, and I feel a weakness that I cannot explain."

Simon examined the large red stain dripping down the front of her gown. "You have lost a great deal of blood. Where were you going—do you remember?"

Catherine furrowed her brow in concentration, desperate to make sense of the confusion that was swirling in her head. *The mayor and Charles had left the house. The fire! That was it. The fire. They were to see the King.* Splinters of memory began to crystallize. "I…I think I was going to the hospital to help."

Simon reached into the medical kit and retrieved the needle and stitching thread. He looked for the source of the blood that was dripping from her temple. "I'll have to stitch the wound, Catherine," he whispered apologetically. "It will hurt." Catherine steeled herself as he gently brushed the hair from her face, exposing a deep gash in her hairline. "Can you hold steady?"

"I'll try, Simon," she whispered. "I'll try."

Simon stroked her hair tenderly once more, and stared at the wound with an aching compassion for the pain he was about to inflict. He threaded the needle, and then gathered the wound together. He took one fiery stab. Catherine flinched, but did not cry out. He took another, then one more. Tears rolled down her cheeks, but still, she was silent. Again and again he drew needle through flesh, six stitches in all. When at last he had finished, Catherine fought the urge to pass out. "We must get you home," worried Simon.

A blinding flash and sudden explosion near the base of the city wall shook the ground, startling them all. Simon and Fitch looked in alarm toward Newgate.

"Ahhh, God, tha's it, nae," whispered Fitch, staring at the imminent danger that now lay before his very eyes, for the driving winds had finally carried the showers of flaming detritus over the city walls. The flames settled upon a row of thatched roof cottages just down the lane from where they sat. The thatch instantly exploded into a scorching fire, sending showers of sparks further down the lane.

"What was that?" asked Catherine, bewildered once more. The entirety of the row was now on fire. Pandemonium raged in the adjacent lanes as the people began to pour from their homes, screaming for help.

"We must get you back to Bealeton House—we must warn your family," urged Simon, watching the flames jump from home to home before his eyes. He was incredulous at the sight. "'Tis time. The winds have turned. The fire has jumped the wall and come to the West End. They will need to retreat, nae."

A sudden realization crystalized in her thoughts. "Simon, your cottage! Hawthorne Lane is nearby. Your research—all your papers!" In her panic, she tried to rise. Simon held her by the shoulders, trying to keep her calm. "Your work—we must save it!" Catherine fought off the hands that restrained her. "We must go!" she cried, trying to stand.

Simon held her down. "Stop! My research *is* safe, Catherine. Father Hardwicke gave his permission. My work is at the hospital. He has it all."

Uncomprehending, she struggled to free herself. "We must go!"

Simon held her close in his arms. He tipped her chin up to focus her attentions. "Look at me, Catherine, my papers, my research…" She stopped fighting and stared into his eyes. "…it is safe. It is *all* safe."

"I don't understand."

"I bound it all in crates last night before I went back to the hospital, in fear that the fire would indeed cross the wall. Father Hardwicke knows the whole of my inquiries. My research was the reason *why* he sent me to Wells to attend to his brother last year. Father Hardwicke knows everything, Catherine, and he understands *why* I did what I did. I was allowed to store the entirety of my research in a storeroom next to his office in the administration building. It is as safe as can be." He watched as tears of sheer relief sprang to her eyes. "We must get you back to Bealeton House."

Simon rose and looked through the escaping crowds up and down the lane. He shook his head. "Aye, there's nary a coach to be had." Resolute, he mounted the horse and held his hand down for her. "Help Lady Catherine, will you, Mr. Fitch?"

"Aye, sir, an' I'll be right behind ye."

Fitch gently helped Catherine to her feet. She clasped Simon's hand. Fitch knitted his fingers together to form a step, and then hoisted her up to the bare back of the horse. She clung to Simon and, laying her head upon his broad back, tried to resist the sleep that threatened to overwhelm her once more. Simon clicked his teeth and they began to thread their way slowly through the fleeing crowds toward Bealeton House.

CHAPTER ELEVEN

Bealeton House
St. James Parish, London
3 September 1666
9:30am

Viola was frantic. She had not moved an inch from the window, watching instead the fearful glow over the city grow ever stronger as the desperate night slid into another day. The thick scent of smoke had grown stronger by the hour. The haze had completely obliterated the morning sun, dimming the mansion to near darkness. With her heart in her throat, she sensed the fire drawing closer, yet she had no word of Catherine, Charles, or Cecil. She could hardly contain the fear roiling her normally idle contemplations.

Viola reached into the embroidery bag at her feet, and tried to thread a needle by the pale candlelight, but her nerves were shot. She was trembling from head to toe. Tears sprang to her eyes as she sat alone in the vast gathering room, wondering what she would save from the home she loved, the home she had poured her heart into. Casting her eyes toward the landing of the mansion's grand oak and marble staircase, her gaze fell upon the towering Peter Lely oil painting, surrounded by a thick, carved golden frame. She'd had the painting of Alvyn, Catherine and Charles commissioned not two years before. Her brother had complained good-naturedly at the expense, but she had been prescient, for the painting was the last likeness captured of her brother before his death. A wistful ache stabbed at her heart. *It is truly magnificent.*

The portrait's astonishing depth of tone, the richness of color and sheer elegance at the hand of the king's much-admired court painter captured the only family she had. It hung majestically in the landing of the staircase for all to admire. In the painting, Sir Alvyn sat in a gold-leafed chair, resplendent in his luxurious crimson waistcoat and white periwig, with Catherine and Charles standing behind him dressed in their most formal clothes. Viola caught her breath each time she gazed upon the painting, for Lely had captured so perfectly the youthful beauty of her niece and nephew, and her brother's merry eyes shining with pride. *'Tis the one true memory of Alvyn I have left.* The sharp pang of his loss caught her once more by surprise. *Nae, if she had to, she would indeed run through fire to save that painting.*

A soft rustle of skirts caught Viola's attention. "Thought ye might like a good, 'ot sip o' tea, Milady," said Gussie Crawdor, the abbey's head cook, rising early for the morning chores. Gussie stopped a moment and cocked an eyebrow at Viola's gown. "Ye've nae been to yer bedchamber this night?" she asked in disbelief, setting down a full tea tray. The hot liquid gurgled and steamed from the spout as she poured. Viola tore her eyes from the window long enough to gratefully take a cup of the strong brew.

"I've been unable to sleep, or indeed even leave the window since they've been gone." Viola looked again through the glass and shook her head in disbelief. "'Tis incomprehensible to think upon the measure of this calamity, Gussie." Viola pointed to the jagged, yellow flames glowing beneath the billowing black clouds over the eastern skyline. "Look there—why, t'was but a mere puff of smoke when first I looked upon it."

Gussie looked through the leaded panes and caught her breath at the ominous glow and the immense clouds of smoke rising above the city. "Would ye like me t' rouse Archie? Perhaps we should return to the Abbey, Milady," she mused aloud.

"The mayor has given his assurance that we are in no danger," Viola snapped, far more harshly than she intended.

"Aye, Milady," nodded Gussie. "I'll not mention it again," she murmured softly. Gussie fell silent and turned toward the window, staring out at the threatening sky.

Viola sighed. "I meant no offense, Gussie." On the carved mantelpiece, a small marble clock chimed softly in the quiet stillness of the mansion.

"None taken, Milady," smiled Gussie, her sensible presence a soothing balm to Viola's high-strung temperament.

"I fear that I am more on edge than I thought," said Viola. "I suppose I shall have to send notes 'round to the guests with our regrets. The wedding will have to be postponed. I should have done it yesterday, just as Mr. Pepys advised." She sighed. "'T'was foolish of me to think we could frolic on as though the danger were only happening inside the city walls." Viola moved a scroll back chair closer, and patted the upholstered seat that had been hand-embroidered in her beloved peacock pattern. "Sit and have some tea, Gussie. Keep me company."

Gussie eased her ample bulk into the chair and poured herself a cup. "Don't mind if I do, Milady." She slipped a sliver of candy sugar into the hot brew and stirred. The silver spoon clinked quietly against the side of the delicate porcelain basin. "'Tis been quite a year, hasn't it, nae?"

Viola turned away and stared at her reflection in the window. She hardly recognized herself. She and Gussie had forged an entirely new relationship during the plague confinement. She found she rather enjoyed it.

Desperate pounding at the front door startled them both. They instantly arose and rushed toward the entrance hall as Simon burst through the door, an unconscious Catherine gathered in his arms. Viola gasped at the sight of the rough stitches, the blood that matted Catherine's hair and stained her gown.

"What's happened, Simon?!" she cried out.

"There's been an accident with the carriage, Lady Hardwicke. Catherine's had a blow to the head…"

Viola cried out in alarm. She squinted her eyes and looked closer, bewildered. "Where are her shoes?" she blurted.

"...and been robbed," he said, his lips set in a grim line.

"Oh, dear God!" Viola cried. Gussie set her feet, bracing herself to catch Viola, for she was positive a swoon was imminent, but to her surprise, Viola gathered her skirts and her thoughts, and took charge.

"Follow me, Simon, we've a bed chamber just at the top of the stairs," said Viola, turning toward the marble steps dimly lit by flickering candle sconces.

"I'll ring for Jane, Milady," said Gussie, hastening belowstairs. "And bring ye a basin of water and some fresh linens. A clean dressing gown, too," she called over her shoulder.

"Aye," said Simon, grimly following Viola up the darkened staircase into a spacious guest chamber. He set Catherine upon the bedstead, laying her head gently on the pillow. Viola looked down at Catherine with grave concern.

"Will she live, Simon?" Worry etched deeply upon her face, Viola could not take her eyes from Catherine lying in the bed so very still, her skin as pale as the fine Holland linens that dressed the feather-stuffed mattress. "I...I don't think I could bear it."

"She will, Lady Hardwicke. With rest, she will indeed soon recover."

Viola pulled a chair next to the bed. "I dare not leave her side."

Before she could sit, Simon gently took hold of her arm and led Viola away from the bedside to the window. Looking out to the swelling plumes of smoke that obscured the faint wash of dawn, he spoke quietly. "I fear there is trouble ahead." She looked up at him in alarm, searching his worried countenance for the slightest jot of reassurance. She found none. "The fires have now crossed the city wall. If the winds shift further toward the West End," He paused, "Bealeton House may be in danger."

CHAPTER TWELVE

nother!" shouted Charles, standing at the head of the fire line in the very midst of the infernos that raged around them. His muscles burned, his eyes were raw and red, even his throat and lungs were scorched from the unceasing smoke and ash—yet after so many others had succumbed to despair, he would not quit.

"Hand me another!" Charles shouted over the thunderous roar, grabbing a leather bucket from the man next to him. He threw the water onto the blaze, and then shoved a lank of straggled red curls from his eyes with the back of his wrist. Though he was covered in soot, his skin burned from the intense heat, his muscles cramped from exhaustion, he still would not quit. Another bucket was thrust into his calloused, bloodied hands. He threw the contents into the burning building. "Again!"

Wiping the cinders and sweat beads from his face, Charles stopped a moment and cast a glance down the lane in disbelief. The devastation was incomprehensible. And yet, though he ached for the profound shock and loss for all those around him, there was something else. Somewhere buried deep inside was a tiny seed of pride to have stood shoulder to shoulder with the Duke of York as the Duke took charge of fighting the fires. *For this one moment, he felt as though he had stepped into his father's shoes.* Upon the Duke's orders, Charles had commandeered willing souls enough to organize three fire lines sending buckets full of water from the Thames up the lanes, one man to the next. King Charles II had even joined the line fighting the blazes that seemed to explode by the minute. *Aye, the crowd loved their Monarch all the more for it,* thought Charles, still awed by the presence of the man who fought to restore the monarchy from the despised Oliver Cromwell just six years before. A sudden crack as a flaming timber fell from the roof of the smithy and smashed into the lane, jerking Charles' attention back to the fire.

"Again!" he cried out.

"Er'e you are, lad!" shouted the blacksmith standing next to Charles, his voice muted over the deafening roar of the flames that shot from the windows of his forge. Charles grabbed the sloshing bucket and passed it on, then turned back and grabbed another. "'Tis like pissin' inta' th' sea, it is," cried the blacksmith, watching in complete despair as flames and smoke billowed from his doorway. Within moments, the entire building was consumed.

"Leave it!" shouted a weary Charles. "Stop the line—there's nothing left to save! Step back!"

"No!" cried the blacksmith. "NO! I'll not go! The smithy! It's me entire life, it is!" He raced down the line desperately grabbing at all the buckets he could hold. He ran back and threw the water into the inferno. "I'll not go! I'll not leave until it burns to the ground!" He turned for another bucket, but the line had stopped. An eerie silence had descended over the lane. Nothing but the forlorn sound of crackling of sparks and timbers collapsing into the ruins could be heard. The men and women on the line stared wordlessly at the blacksmith, their shoulders slumped in defeat. There would be no more water.

"Mon Dieu."

The exhausted crowd whipped their heads toward a pitiable woman standing alone by the side of the lane, quietly staring at the incomprehensible destruction. She carried a wooden spoon in one hand and clutched at her cloak with the other. *"Mon Dieu,"* she moaned once again.

"Er'e nae! What's she sayin?" shouted a man from the back of a crowd that had begun to form around her.

"Jaysus, she's a damnable Frenchie, she is!" cried another, shoving closer to get a better look.

"Tha' Frenchie's hidin' somethin'!" shouted another man standing near the woman, pointing to a bulge beneath her cloak. "Look at 'er!"

"'Tis a firebomb!" screeched an old woman. "A firebomb, I tell ye!"

The crowd gave a collective gasp. "Firebomb!" they screamed, the mere word striking terror into the hearts of the exhausted congregation. Powerless to stop the fires and terrified at the thought that foreigners were exacting their revenge for the war, the men in the crowd instantly descended like rabid dogs upon the Frenchwoman. Enraged, the mob lunged at her, knocking her to the ground. She cried out, grasping tightly to her cloak.

"Je ne comprends pas!" she screamed, desperately trying to fight them off. *"Arrete, s'il vous plait! Arrete!"* The wooden spoon clattered against the cobblestones. *"Je ne comprends pas!"*

Charles elbowed his way into the crowd. "Stop! She doesn't understand!" he shouted. A man grabbed both his arms and held him back. "She says she doesn't understand!" Charles cried once more, struggling to evade the binding grasp.

High above the mob that held the woman down, a dagger glittered in the smithy's dwindling firelight. A deep voice cried out, "Damnable foreigners!" as the dagger disappeared from sight. The woman screamed in agony as the sharp blade swiftly found its mark, again and again.

Charles broke free. "No! Stop! *STOP!*" he screamed, as he shoved his way through the crowd. Charles raced toward the woman who now lay on the ashen-covered lane in a widening pool of blood. He threw both hands over the deep slashes, in a desperate attempt to quell the blood that pulsed from her wounds. She turned to Charles with anguished, searching eyes and whispered quietly, *"Je ne comprends pas."* The crowd gathered in close. Forming a circle around the dying woman, they fell silent. After a moment, her head rolled softly to the side.

A man dressed in soot-covered rags backed slowly away. He raised a vengeful fist that clutched the bloody knife. "Damnable foreigners! Kill 'em all!" he screamed. The dagger clattered dully onto the cobblestones. The man turned and ran from the lane, his soft footsteps fading away in the shocked silence. The crowd gasped and drew back in fear as Charles unlaced the cowlings around the woman's neck. He thrust a fist into her cloak and grabbed hold of something. He stood and faced the incensed mob.

"A chicken!" he shouted, thrusting the pitiful bird high for all to see. A plump, yellow roaster squawked in feeble protest. "The woman concealed a chicken!" he sputtered. "A chicken!" His voice cracked in fury. Charles stood and faced the woman's tormentors, angry beyond measure. "What justice is it that an innocent woman standing alone on the lane should be tried without a hearing, convicted without a jury—and murdered in cold blood without cause?" he shouted to the feral mob. "And for what, I ask you? For *what?!*" He took a deep breath to calm himself. One by one, the villagers stepped back in horror from the dead woman, shaken by the demented thirst for blood and revenge that had seized their minds. Charles looked down the now deserted lane. "Who among you knows the man who ran from here?" The silent crowd, as one, looked down in shame to the blackened cobblestones. A few women crossed themselves in prayer. No one spoke. "No man is above the law, even in desperate times!" cried an impassioned Charles.

In the quiet of the crackling flames, a hollow clatter of hoof beats approached from the rear. Heads turned to see the Duke galloping toward them, his horse rearing and pawing in the air at the destruction surrounding the fire line.

"Master Abbott," shouted the Duke, wheeling his horse in a circle, searching above the crowd.

"Aye, sir!" called Charles. He took a step forward. The Duke pulled his horse up short, as it snorted and bucked at the bridle's pull.

"The winds turned to the west early this morning. There is now a desperate need for more fire lines outside the wall at Ludgate," called the Duke. "If these westerly winds hold, Whitehall will be directly in the fire's path and we will be forced to take drastic measures." He stopped a moment, knowing the panic his next words would cause. "If we are unable to hold the Ludgate line, all homes and shops to the west will be destroyed using gun powder enough to form a firebreak and save the palace!" The fearful crowd cried out in contemplation of the impending disaster. The Duke leaned down to Charles. "Are you able to organize men enough to assist in the Ludgate fire lines?"

"Yes, sir!" A sudden realization sent a shiver of fear down his spine. *Bealeton House lies to the west.* He faced the Duke square on. "I am, indeed."

CHAPTER THIRTEEN

"THE VERY COBBLES GLOWED WITH A FIERY REDNESS SO
AS NO HORSE OR MAN ABLE TO TREAD UPON THEM."
~ SAMUEL PEPYS

City of Westminster
Middlesex, England
4 September 1666
5:03 am

Cecil fought through the panicked crowds on Fleet Street, working his way toward Bealeton House amid the screams of the terrified souls, the searing heat and the burning flakes of fire that fell like black snow around him, illuminating the dawn as though it were midday. Just as one parish burned to the ground, the relentless winds carried the fire on to the next. *Aye'n, no one is safe from these diabolical flames.* In the midst of the raging chaos and confusion, he had become separated from Charles sometime during the first hours, and had not seen the lad since. Samuel, too, had parted ways to command fire lines down at the river. Cecil, like so many others, had simply roamed the turbulent city, joining the fire lines wherever he found them, wherever extra hands were desperately needed. It had been a long, dreadful siege and although the devastation was not yet over, he now could take no more. It felt as though the cataclysm would never end. He was beginning his third day fighting the fires. Nearly three days stealing sleep when he could, laying his head upon piled up rags or a patch of grass for scant minutes at a time. Nearly three days of sheer hell on earth.

He was not a young man. Every bone in his body ached. His back hurt. A sudden pain shot through his left arm. As he stretched to work out the kink, a young woman clutching tightly to the hand of a small child banged awkwardly into his shoulder. He groaned and stepped back, wincing. The soot-laden cloth bundle she carried on her back fell dully to the ground in a puff of ash, spilling the few pieces of clothing she had stuffed inside and a loaf of bread onto the filthy lane. In mute disbelief at the sight of her meager possessions kicked about and crushed by people racing to escape the inferno, she sagged slowly to her knees. Exhausted tears streamed down her face. The sleepy little boy stared up at him, wordlessly blinking saucer blue eyes. Cecil's soft heart melted.

"Ahhhh, there, there, Miss. Don't cry, nae," he said, retrieving the loaf of bread from the ground. He brushed the ashes off and tucked the bread under his arm, and then ran into the fleeing crowds to gather her clothing. He rolled the young woman's belongings into a small bundle, then put it all back into the pack and tied the rope knot tighter. He handed the pack to her. "There 'tis, Miss, tidy and true," he said, encouragingly. "All's the better, nae." He tilted his head in thought, and then reached deep into the pocket of his breeches. Cecil winked. He leaned down to the boy and pulled out a hard chip of boiled sugar wrapped in crinkly oilpaper. "All's the better, indeed," he whispered. He handed the boy the small bite of candy. In that single moment, in the midst of the unending sadness and terrible ruin that surrounded them all, the little boy smiled.

The young woman wiped her eyes and rose to her feet. "I'm grateful to ye, sir." She took a deep breath, and then hoisted the pack onto her back, taking hold of her son's hand once again. Cecil watched them disappear into the turbulent crowd. It was a small moment of kindness in the midst of such unrelenting despair, yet he felt terribly sad. His emotions were roiling on the surface. In his fatigue, his heart ached for all that had been destroyed, for the incomprehensible and profound losses to all in his beloved city. Weariness weighing heavily upon his chest, Cecil turned and trudged once more toward home.

CHAPTER FOURTEEN

St. Bartholomew's Hospital
Smithfield Parish, London
4 September 1666
5:21 am

Father Thomas Hardwicke needed air. His head ached. His lungs were filled with the overwhelming stench of burned flesh. The unending cries and moans of the injured, the sheer amount of the wounded crowded into every inch of his hospital dulled his spirits and shook his faith in God. Called from his cloistered administration offices during the first desperate hours of the fire by overwhelmed physicians to assist the wounded and dying, Father Hardwicke had performed more death ministrations in the past three days than he had performed in his entire ten years as Chief Administrator of hospital. The very walls of the vast, timbered hall of St. Bartholomew's had at last begun to close in upon him.

The old priest leaned down and laid his hands gently upon the forehead of yet another victim, a small boy of about five years. Moved to tears, he gazed at the dead child, lying still and so terribly alone on the pallet. *The pitiable lad had no one to grieve for him.* Dressed in his heavy, formal surplice, the cloistered, stinking air of the hospital began to make him feel faint. His hands began to shake. Father Hardwicke sat on the edge of the rope pallet. A thick, golden cross suspended from a gold chain around his neck knocked into his anointing vessel, spilling several drops of the oil onto the rough cotton sheeting that covered the boy. Mercifully inhaling the oil's spicy wafts of orange blossom, rose, cinnamon, jasmine, musk, civet and wooded ambergris that had been custom blended for King

Charles I, even the beloved, sacred fragrance could not revive his aching soul. He sprinkled the thick oil droplets over the boy and sighed. "Into your hands, O merciful Savior, we commend your young servant. Receive him into the arms of your mercy, into the blessed rest of everlasting peace, and into the glorious company of the saints in light. Amen," he whispered, as he covered the boy's face with the cloth. Father Hardwicke stood, his heart—nae his very soul—shattered by the vastness of death and ruination around him. *He could take no more.*

It was well before dawn's rising when he stepped into the still turbulent street outside the hospital. He no longer knew day from night, the torches in the hospital having been kept lit when the choking smoke outside dimmed the interior to darkness. Though there was the barest trace of daylight, any hopes for fresh air were dashed when the pungent, choking clouds of smoke overwhelmed his senses. Father Hardwicke thought briefly of turning back, but could not bring himself to enter the hospital again. Though the thick, drifting haze was dense, he sought to clear his head by taking a walk around the hospital to the administration offices at the rear. As he turned the corner of Bartholomew's Close, he was unnerved to see the fire's foreboding glow under a tremendous swath of black smoke that hung over the distant city center. *Our God has shown us his glory and his majesty, and on this day we hear his voice from the fire.* For a disorienting, almost comical moment, Father Hardwicke wondered what God could possibly be trying to say. Bumped and jostled from all sides, he forced his way through the chaotic, shouting rabble conveying all manner of wounded into the hospital, then turned onto the narrow lane behind the stone structure. Mercifully, the crowd began to thin, before finally dissipating altogether. *At last a moment of peace.* He stopped to pull a long clay pipe from the pocket of his surplice, and then struck a sharp flint, setting flame to the snuff-filled bowl. Inhaling deeply, Father Hardwicke felt the tension in his shoulders slowly ease off as he leaned against the wall and blew a lazy puff of smoke into the blackened air. He watched for a moment as the pale gray tendrils swirled into the charcoal ash, creating an ethereal miasma of smut. After several minutes of contemplation and prayer, he tamped out the pipe, then turned and walked on.

Crossing an alley to the rarely used rear entrance of the administration offices Father Hardwicke paused at the doorway. His thick, golden neck chain glittered under the flickering flame of a single oil lantern that illuminated the entrance. *He did not know if he had the strength to go back in.* Behind him, he heard footsteps. He reached for the iron latch and jiggled it, but in the confusion of the fire, the padlock had been left in place. He reached for a leather cord on his belt that held several thick keys to the administration buildings. The footsteps grew closer. He turned to see who approached, but the dawn's light had not yet reached in the dark, empty alley. He had an odd, deeply unsettling sense of danger. He fumbled for the iron padlock key. The footsteps grew closer. He looked back once more. His heart began to pound.

"Who is there?!" he cried out.

From the shadows a dark figure suddenly lunged at him, grabbing hold of the golden cross. He felt the vicious yank at his neck, and then a crushing blow as something hard cracked into the back of his skull. His knees buckled. Father Hardwicke felt himself sag to the ground at the doorway. In the smudging darkness, the thief disappeared back down the alley and slipped into the crowd.

CHAPTER FIFTEEN

St. James Parish
London, England
4 September 1666
4:57 pm

A plaintive raven's screech next to his head startled Cecil from a deep slumber. Lying under an elegant line of trees in St. James Park, he had no idea how long he had slept on the soft, velvety patch of grass that had been far too tempting to pass by. It felt as though he had slept for weeks. Cecil sat up in the fading light of day and squinted through the dense smoke, unable for once to admire the park's formal gardens that had been redesigned as homage to the elaborate landscapes of French palaces so revered by King Charles II. He knew the fires were drawing ever closer. Cecil sighed and arose, gathering his cloak. In his exhaustion, Cecil caught the toe of his boot on an exposed root and stumbled. Throwing his hands down to the dirt to catch his fall, he sank to the ground to rest another moment, staring in disbelief at the monumental scale of the disaster now unfolding over the entire city. To his right, heavy drifts of smoke hung thick over the lake obscuring his view of the Royal Swans, a sight that had always soothed his soul. To his left, the hatchways of the aviary had been opened and through the floating soot and ash, he could see the forlorn cages, now barren of the King's vast collection of shimmering blue peacocks. Cecil sighed. Please God that the creatures have all found safe refuge.

Lifting his gaze above the treetops, he saw the black, churning clouds of ash that now blew unchecked over the West End, dimming the lush, autumnal colors of the park's foliage.

It was a singularly depressing sight that weighed heavily on his thoughts. The smoke brought stinging tears to his eyes, though he could not say whether the tears were from the ashes or the profound sorrow that overcame him at the sight of it all. He could barely breathe. He was exhausted. He took a handkerchief from his pocket and wiped his brow. He was sweating heavily. He stared at the white linen, now streaked with filth and felt an unaccustomed heaviness upon his heart. An ominous dread settled deep in his bones as he contemplated the course he now faced. *He had been so very wrong.* He had badly misjudged the enormity of the peril three days ago. He had given Viola false hope that they were safe from the fires. *They were now most assuredly not.* He had seen with his own eyes that there was no place to safely hide their most treasured possessions, for even the vast courtyard of St. Paul's Cathedral, as others had desperately run to with their valuables, had been rendered to ruin. The magnificent structure had burned to the ground in the night, the fire being so hot that the lead roof had melted and poured down the surrounding lanes of Ludgate Hill. They would now only have time enough to gather a few valuables and retreat immediately to the Abbey. *Would she er'e forgive my overly blithesome counsel?* He dreaded facing Viola, for he feared the ensuing panic his edict would cause. Cecil unfurled his handkerchief and reluctantly stood, knotting the cloth around his face as he turned for home.

❧

Catherine opened her eyes to a strange, disorienting feeling. In the faded light, she stared at the room's hand-stenciled botanical wallpaper. The delicately painted oranges that hung from arching tree branches looked not at all familiar. Her fingers played upon the thin, ice blue stripe that finished the sheetings edge. For a moment, she did not recognize where she was. Catherine threw the crisp, woven bed linens aside and swung her feet to the floor, feeling a sharp ache at her temple. Memories of the accident came flooding back. She instinctively reached up and touched the stitches in wonderment. *How long have I slept?* She looked closely at the small, ebony table clock beside the bedstead, and then rose, pulling on a thick, velvet robe that had been placed at the end of the bed. She walked slowly to the paned window. A moment of dizzying weakness overcame her. She set her hand upon a carved armoire to steady herself, and then moved the tapestry draperies aside. She caught her breath, for although she knew by the clock that it was not yet night, it was nearly black outside from the vast amount of smoke that filled the air. She could scarcely believe the billowing clouds that obscured the lane. The thick smell of smoke was frightening, even inside the room. An overwhelming panic clutched at her stomach. The latch on her door clicked softly. She turned to see Viola entering the room, with Jane, carrying a basin of cool water and a thick cloth over her arm, following close behind.

"Why are you out of bed, Catherine?" said Viola, fretting. "You must rest, you've had quite the injury to your head."

Catherine threw the draperies wide and faced her aunt. "The fire is coming this way!" she cried.

Viola stopped short. "Nonsense. It is just the winds blowing the smoke. Cecil gave his assurance that the fire will not reach the West End."

"No! We must leave," Catherine said, urgently. Visions of the fire jumping the London wall flooded back into her consciousness. "I have seen it—the whole of the city is in flames. You cannot imagine the destruction—we cannot stay!" She threw open the doors to the armoire. It was empty. She turned to Viola. "Where are my clothes?"

"Upstairs, in your room."

"Jane, please bring me a gown." Jane slipped out of the room. Catherine composed herself. She looked once again out the window, and then turned once more to Viola. "The Abbey." Her voice rose in intensity. "We must retreat to the Abbey!"

"Shhhh, Catherine, you are overwrought," she soothed, leading Catherine back to the bedstead. "We cannot retreat."

Catherine fought her grasp. "But, the smoke! Can you not smell it? The fire is coming this way. We *must* leave London!" The dread she felt was now palpable. Her head was pounding.

Viola led Catherine back to the bedstead and spoke firmly. "Catherine, you must listen to me, now. We have no means of travel. The carriage has been destroyed and one horse has been stolen. The cook's cart is out supplying the firelines with food from the kitchen, and Simon has taken the remaining horse to look for Charles and Cecil who are still out fighting the fires," she paused. "Until they return, there is simply nothing else to be done." She patted the feather mattress. "I insist that you return to bed and rest."

Before Catherine could mount further protest, the heavy front door slammed one floor below. Startled, Catherine and Viola ran from the room to the gallery and looked down into the entrance hall where Cecil stood, his shoulders slumped in exhaustion. Beads of sweat glistened on his brow. In the faded light, his pallor looked an unearthly shade of gray. Unwinding his filthy cravat to open his collar wide, he sank to a settee by the doorway, and dropped his head back against the wall for a scant moment of rest.

"Cecil!" cried Viola, gathering her skirts. She hurried down the stairs. "Three days and no word! I've been beside myself!"

Catherine watched from the railing as he stood once more to take Viola into his arms. He held her tight, laying his head gently atop hers. In that tender moment, time stood still. Catherine descended the stairs, setting her hand to the wall for balance. As she drew closer, Catherine could see the exhausted tears in Cecil's eyes. She saw the dirt and ash that sullied his clothes and blackened his face. She saw the bleak desolation that seemed to have taken hold of his very being. He lifted his head and stepped back, taking Viola's hands into his. Halfway down the stairs, Catherine felt dizzy. She sat down upon a step and watched the mayor deliver the devastating news.

"My dear, I must beg your forgiveness," he confessed. "The fires are upon us, nae." He could not look at her, such was the guilt that overcame his sensibilities. "I was wrong," he said, choking back emotion. "We must abandon Bealeton House, immediately."

Viola gasped. "No, Cecil!"

"I know you do not wish to leave, but Viola, the entire city now lies in unthinkable ruin. The fires have jumped the wall. The West End is no longer protected. The winds this hour drive the fires straight toward us."

"We have no means of escape!" she breathed, suddenly grasping the enormity of the situation.

"What?" Cecil looked up to Catherine on the stairway, shocked by her bandaged head. "Catherine, my dear! You've been hurt!" He turned to Viola. "What has happened in my absence?"

"There was an accident and the carriage has been destroyed. One of the horses was stolen." Viola quickly ticked off the remaining list of complications on her pale fingertips. "Catherine has been injured, and the men have not yet returned with the horsecart. The wedding has been cancelled and the London staff has been dismissed to attend to their families. Simon has taken the remaining horse and has gone to find Charles." She turned to him in shock. "Until they return, Cecil, we have no way to return to Stockbridge and the Abbey."

"I am well enough, Aunt Viola," insisted Catherine, composed once more. "I agree with Uncle, we *must* be ready when Simon returns. We will pack what we can and prepare to leave as soon as possible," said Catherine as she rose and headed toward her third floor suite.

Cecil concurred. "Viola, you and I shall do the same. The Abbey staff will have to gather their things, as well. With just one cart, we all must take only the most valuable, the most irreplaceable items and leave the rest behind." Catherine looked back to Viola, fearing that she would panic. To her complete shock, Viola seemed more than calm and capable.

"Gussie will organize the staff belowstairs," said Viola. She stopped a moment, gazing at the mansion's irreplaceable treasures that she had spent years collecting, and then lifted her chin and squared her shoulders. She faced Cecil. "There is just one thing I beg of you to save." She turned and pointed to the painting of Sir Alvyn on the stairwell landing.

❧

Incessant winds swirled through the lanes as Simon fought his way through a staggering amount of fiery debris toward the fire's perimeter. Every building within miles was either burning or had burned to the ground. His cottage on Hawthorn Lane had burned. *Everything had burned.* Papers, cinders, even bits of clothing and wood tumbled every which way in the howling winds that blew through the thick, fouled air. He hardly knew which direction to turn, the perimeter having spread farther than he could see through the dense smoke. His horse began to snort wildly, struggling to clear the ashes and debris from his nostrils. Simon dismounted and threw off his cloak. He ripped his shirt off, and then wrapped the fabric around the horse's face, knotting the arms together to keep the sparking ashes at bay. He stepped back and wiped his stinging eyes, made wet and coarse from the thick, gritty smoke, and then tore a piece of his linen tunic into a length of cloth and wound it around his own face. Donning the cloak once more, Simon remounted and pulled the reins.

At the River Fleet, Simon led the horse high upon the bank. Drawing the leathers up sharply, he gasped and stared at the uncontrollable devastation that now engulfed the entire city. He wound the cloth tighter around his face. Looking first northward, and then to the south, he was at a complete loss. He had no idea where to begin to look for Charles. Though thousands of fiery flakes and ash rained down upon him, pelting his face and hands with tiny sparks and the acrid smell of burning hair stung his nostrils, Simon felt nothing but an overwhelming dread, for the fires had burned everything as far as he could see. The Old Bailey, the Royal Exchange, St. Paul's Cathedral were all destroyed. *He could not imagine, even in his worst nightmares, the vast amount of destruction he now lay witness to.* Simon grasped the reins tighter, then kicked the horse and rode on.

The lanes to the northeast and Smithfield beyond were oddly dark and deserted, save the few citizens who remained, keening over the desolate, smoking ruins of their homes. Simon approached the thick, fortified wall of Aldersgate. He jumped to the dirt and, lashing the horse to a post, raced up the narrow, circular ragstone staircase, its ancient treads worn low in the middle from centuries of regimental soldiers climbing to the top of the deserted gatehouse. He unlatched the planked door to the rooftop and pushed it wide. His boots left pale imprints upon the ashes as he skidded across to the edge of the stone bulwark. In the unearthly silence, Simon peered through an archer's loophole to take the measure of the fire's perimeter. He gazed with dread at a silent, apocalyptic wall of black smoke rising far, far above London. The flames now stretched for miles upon miles in every direction. *Dear God, the entirety of London has been leveled to ashes.* Simon caught his breath. *It will be nigh' impossible to find Charles.*

A violent series of explosions to the west caught his eye. Just beyond the brilliant showers of sparks, soaring flames and jarring concussions of the explosions he could see the faint silhouette of Whitehall Palace. Setting his hands to the stone ledge to steady himself, Simon fully understood. *They intend to save the palace by setting firebreaks in the path of the inferno.* A sudden panic overwhelmed his thoughts. *Bealeton House is in that path.* Simon bolted back down the narrow stone steps and out to the lane. Throwing his leg over the saddle, Simon kicked the horse and wheeled his mount eastward in a desperate race toward St. James.

CHAPTER SIXTEEN

"I WAS NOT ABLE TO PASSE THROUGH ANY OF THE NARROW
STREETES, BUT KEPT THE WIDEST; THE GROUND AND AIR, SMOAKE
AND FIERY VAPOUR CONTINU'D SO INTENSE, THAT MY HAIRE
WAS ALMOST SING'D AND MY FEETE UNSUFFERABLY SURFEATED."
~ SIR JOHN EVELYN

Bealeton House
St. James Parish, London
4 September 1666
8:47 pm

A violent, thunderous string of cannonades in the near
distance shook the walls of the mansion as Catherine
descended the staircase carrying a small bag. Jagged cracks began
to scar the stairwell plaster, spreading upwards. Chunks of debris
fell from the chimney flue down to the grate. Billowing clouds of
ash swelled out in waves onto the tapestry carpet that lay before
the marble hearth, dulling the colored woolen threads. At the
jolting explosions, Catherine grabbed at the wall for balance
and looked to Cecil in alarm as he passed on his way up to the
landing. He was dragging a heavy wooden footstool.

"What was that?" she asked, alarmed at the thundering fusillades.

Cecil shook his head. "I'm afraid I don't know, my dear.
Perhaps t'was the ales of the mighty Black Eagle brewhouse
blowing high to the heavens. Alcohol is quite flammable, you
know," he winked, seeking to ease her fears. "More's the pity."

Catherine gave a rueful smile. "Where is Mr. Crawdor?
Should we not wait to remove the painting until Charles and
Simon have returned, Uncle? You must be tired. You've not had
proper sleep in days."

"Nonsense, Catherine. I am rested enough. We have no idea when the men will return, and Archie is in the garden burying the Bordeaux—a far more important task at the moment."

"But the painting—the frame is taller than you by half and nearly as wide… Surely you cannot lift it from the wall yourself."

Cecil shot Catherine a withering glance. "I am not as infirm as you may think, my dear." He set the three-legged stool before the painting that hung several feet from the ground and took its measure. "Though perhaps it is a jot larger than I thought," he muttered to himself.

"I did not mean to offend, Uncle" she said, chagrined.

Another series of deafening explosions rattled the mansion's leaded glass windowpanes. Cecil glanced toward the windows and raised an eyebrow. "There goes the Griffin Brewery," he quipped, as he stepped back warily estimating the weight of the massive frame.

Viola appeared at the second floor balcony. "Cecil!" she fussed. "Have a care! Let someone help…"

"Nonsense, Viola," he said, cutting her off. "I'll not hear another word. I'm not some old dallywag incapable of lifting a three-penny stone."

Catherine laughed as she watched Cecil wave Viola away from the heavy oak balustrade like a fusty old hen. He stepped upon the stool and tried to hoist the frame from its mounting hooks. Another sharp pain shot through his left arm. He paused, rubbing his shoulder muscles as he contemplated its heft. It weighed far more than he expected. "Perhaps I should wait, indeed," he murmured. Cecil's plans were interrupted by a cry from the lower hall.

"The cook's cart has returned!" shouted Archie, from the top of the servant's staircase.

"Aye, Archie. Well done," called Cecil.

"I regret to say that only Fitch will stay on, sir. The rest of the men request leave to save their own homes," called Archie, climbing the wooden treads of the main staircase.

Cecil stepped down from the stool. "As they should, Archie. As they should, indeed." Cecil's demeanor suddenly shifted. "There it is, then. Give the men something to eat and a few moments rest. When they are sufficiently refreshed, have them load the cart. We shall all depart thereafter."

"Aye, Milord."

"I'll not leave without Charles," insisted Viola from the balcony. "And, the painting." She was adamant in her determination. "Pack anything you wish into the cart, Cecil, however, I will not leave him—or it—behind."

"We do not know when Charles will return—it may be days, Viola!" Cecil cried, impatiently. "These explosions are meant to stop the fires advance, and they draw nearer by the hour. I insist that we now depart with all speed." He became adamant. "I'll not listen to another word."

"And I'll not leave without Charles," she repeated, firmly setting her hands upon the balustrade.

Cecil shook his head in resignation, knowing he was far, far overmatched.

Incessant pounding at the mansion's door interrupted the argument. Without warning, the door swung wide and Simon ran in, followed by the sound of yet another powerful set of explosions that lit the entire sky ablaze behind him. Catherine raced from the landing down the stairs.

"Simon!" she cried.

Simon took her into his arms, and then, holding her tightly, called up to Viola, still standing on the vast second floor balcony. "I beg your forgiveness for the sudden intrusion, Milady." He nodded to Cecil. "Milord."

"What news, Simon?" asked Cecil, concerned by the abrupt entrance.

"I must be direct, sir," said Simon. "It is time, nae. I have witnessed for myself that the fires have now spread into St. James Parish. The Duke has called in the military. They are setting explosive gunpowder charges to the homes and shops on the east side of the park, and I believe Charles to be with them. It is but a matter of time before they come this way." He hesitated. "You must abandon Bealeton House within the hour." He turned to Catherine. "The cottage has burned to the ground—along with nearly all of London. 'Tis a disaster the likes of which none have 'ere seen in this lifetime."

"Oh, Simon, your cottage!" Catherine cried. "I am so sorry."

"The hospital has thus far been spared. The cottage was let and my belongings are safely away in the hospital's administration building. If we all remain safe, we can ask for nothing more. There are thousands upon thousands who gather at Moorfield's Park with nothing but the clothes on their backs. 'Tis but a direful catastrophe like no other…"

Catherine looked up at Simon and whispered. "I confess… I am afraid."

Simon held her tightly for a moment; gazing deep into her intelligent, gray eyes. Her soft, pale-pink skin glowed in the blazing firelight through the smoked-streaked panes of the front window. He touched her wound with great care. *How he longed to protect her, to confide in her, to share his thoughts—nae, to share his very life with this beautiful creature he held in his arms.* He had absolutely no reservations. *He could not bear to wait another moment.*

Stepping back, he began to unwind the length of rough linen cloth from his neck. He kissed Catherine once more, and then, Simon turned to face the mayor, proffering the cloth with earnest eyes. The mayor took hold of it, thoughtfully fingering the rough, ash-covered fabric. Cecil cocked his head, and then smiled, nodding his assent.

"I suppose there is indeed time enough, my boy."

Instantly grasping the significance of the gesture, Viola cried out and clapped her hands together. She grabbed hold of her skirts and hurried down the stairs to the formal entry. She removed the lace shawl from around her shoulders and held it toward Simon.

"Perhaps you would care to use this, instead?"

"Aye, Lady Hardwicke, I believe we would, indeed," he said, exchanging the filthy linen cloth in Cecil's hands with the ivory-colored lace. Simon stuffed the linen cloth into his tunics. "I am most grateful."

Viola stepped back and stood expectantly next to Cecil, her eyes shining with excitement. Catherine looked from one to the other and then back to Simon again, confusion writ large across her face.

Simon turned to Catherine and took her hands protectively into his own. He leaned in close. "I promised to marry you this night," he whispered. "Though the circumstances have much changed, I pray that you will nonetheless take me now as your husband with a handfasting ceremony."

Tears sprang to Catherine's eyes. "Oh, Simon, yes. Yes! I will indeed marry you," she cried.

He looked to Cecil. "Would you please, as the Lord Mayor of Wells—and my very dear friend—perform the ceremony?"

"T'would be my honour, indeed," said Cecil, rocking back and forth on his heels, his face flushed red with anticipation.

Viola reached into her sleeve and withdrew an embroidered handkerchief. Dabbing her eyes, she reached for a bell on the entry table and rang it. A maid appeared. "Although the London staff have left to attend to their own families, would you please ask those who remain to join us," asked Viola.

"Aye, Milady, I will indeed."

Within minutes, the few remaining staff assembled in the formal hall. At Viola's bidding, two maids lit the iron and crystal candelabras that filled the expansive entrance hall.

Cecil cocked an eyebrow toward Viola. "Considering the circumstances, my dear, you would require candleflame?" The honeyed scent of beeswax began to mix with the thick smoke that filled the air.

"What matter could it possibly make, now, Cecil?" said Viola, dryly. She cast an appreciative eye upon the soft flames that reflected a wavering glow across the black and white marble flooring. "Though unspeakable disaster gather without, I shall *not* be deprived of a romantic wedding ceremony, however small it may be, within this house."

"Aye'n yer right, Milady!" breathed Gussie. "Wait a tick, will ye?" she cried, running to the nearby butler's pantry. "I have somethin' fer ye." In moments, she returned carrying a small bouquet of linen-wrapped ivory roses that had been gathered for the cancelled ceremony in one hand, and an intertwining coronet of the same fragrant roses in the other. Gussie handed the bouquet to Catherine, and then gently set the flowered wreath atop the copper curls that cascaded down Catherine's back, taking great care to avoid the wound. "I had these made fer ye." Catherine touched her fingertips lightly upon the crown of roses and caught her breath. Gussie stepped back and took Archie's hand tightly into hers.

"Thank you, Gussie," breathed Catherine, her eyes glistening with tears, overcome by the love she felt for the woman who had cared for her since the long ago death of her mother, and now, the death of her beloved father.

The mayor stepped between the gleaming candelabras. "Very well, then," he nodded. "Catherine, Simon, please clasp your right hands together."

Simon reached for Catherine's hand and took it tenderly into his own. As the mayor began to wind the lace around their joined hands, the latch on the front door rattled. All heads turned at the sound. Cedric opened the door to an exhausted Charles, backlit by a fearsome, truly fiendish glow. He entered the mansion and stopped short, momentarily confused by the sight of the small gathering. Charles suddenly smiled softly and looked to Simon. "You would marry my sister without my presence?"

Catherine unwound herself from the lace and ran to her brother, hugging him tightly. "Charles, you're safe!"

"I am, though I bear direful news." He turned to face the anxious gathering. "The Duke has ordered a massive firebreak in a last ditch effort to save Whitehall Palace. The soldiers are now blasting homes across the park." Viola gasped and reached for Cecil's hand. "If the firebreak does not hold, they will advance to this side."

"No!" cried Viola. She leaned against Cecil. "There are simply no words for this catastrophe. What's to become of London?"

Charles tried to soften the blow. "I have asked the Duke to spare our street by all available means, and he has consented— but only to the point where it is no longer possible. He looked to Viola, sadness in his eyes. "I cannot promise you that Bealeton House will remain safe. We can only pray, now."

Another spectacular explosion rocked the house, sending the maids screaming as they ducked for cover. Jane turned pale and began to shake with fear. Viola grabbed for Cecil's arm to regain her balance. At the unholy blast, the plaster walls concussed inward, causing the hairline cracks to widen and spread. In the gathering room, a large chunk of masonry broke free and crashed to the floor, scarring deeply into the floorboards. Priceless vases wobbled on their stands then fell to the ground, shattering into hundreds of pieces. Hanging candle chandeliers swung to and fro, their faceted crystal droplets refracting rainbow flashes across the cream-colored walls. Yellowed beeswax spilled from the candleholders as the tremulations settled. Jane ran to collect the broken vases, slicing her finger on the shards of glass that spread wide across the entry hall. She held the gash to her mouth, wincing at the sight of blood. The kitchen maid worked to scrape the spilled wax from the cold marble tiles.

"Leave it," called Viola. The maids looked back in surprise. "Leave it," Viola sighed. "There is no point." The maids quietly returned to the entry. Viola leaned over and whispered to Catherine. "I'm afraid this is not much of a ceremony, my dear."

Catherine gazed at the faces crowding in a half-circle around her. Gussie leaned against Archie, her eyes glistening with pride. It was her beloved Gussie who gave her sweets, bandaged every scraped knee and looked on with fascination at every butterfly, insect and flower she collected as a child. Archie's soft heart showed in every deep wrinkle of his craggy face. She was overcome.

"Aunt Viola, I am surrounded by the people I love most in this world, and I stand with the man I love more than life itself. Though I miss Father terribly, I do not believe I could ask for a more perfect ceremony."

The mayor stepped back between the candelabras. He spoke to Catherine and Simon. "I believe we may have but minutes to spare. Do you wish to continue?" he asked gently.

"Aye, Milord," said Simon, firmly. "We do."

"Yes, Uncle."

"Very well, then. Please join your right hands." The mayor wound the lace twice around their wrists. He faced Simon. "Do you, Simon McKensie, take thee, Lady Catherine Mary Abbott, to be your wedded wife till death you depart?"

He looked to Catherine and smiled. "I do."

"And thereto, do you plight thee your troth."

"I do, indeed," he said, softly.

Cecil faced Catherine.

"And do you, Lady Catherine Mary Abbott, take thee Simon McKensie to be your wedded husband till death you depart?"

"I do."

"And thereto, do you plight thee your troth."

"I do," she whispered, her eyes shining.

The mayor turned to the little gathering. "By virtue of *Sponsalia de Praesenti,* this couple hath declared here and nae that they affirm one to the other as man and wife." He turned to Simon and Catherine. "Be it known to all that in as much as handfasting vows are a legal and valid binding of two souls in matrimony, you will henceforth be known to all as Dr. Simon and Lady Catherine McKensie."

With tears in his eyes, Simon gathered Catherine closely into his arms and, to the maids great, giggling delight, kissed her for just a moment longer than custom would allow. The mayor tactfully cleared his throat. Red-faced, Simon caught himself and stepped back. Deeply embarrassed, Simon fished into his pocket and withdrew the golden timepiece. He held it toward Catherine. "I had this engraved by Master East at the Clockmaker's Company in the Royal Exchange." He turned the watch over. "The watchcase was etched with today's date before the fire altered our plans. I pray that you will accept it as a token of our marriage."

Catherine wiped tears away herself. She took the watch in hand, running her fingers lightly over the engraving. *4 September 1666.* "I would be honored, Simon," she whispered. "Thank you." She stood on her tiptoes and taking his rough, stubbled face in hand, kissed him once more.

Gussie could hardly contain herself. She let out a squeal and a little jump, and then wrapped Catherine in a massive hug. "Aye'n yer father and mother would be proud of ye an' Doctor McKensie," she whispered. "I'm so happy for ye, my lamb."

Viola stepped up and took Simon in a warm embrace. "I'm happy for you both."

As Simon embraced both Charles and Cecil, another violent string of explosions echoed through the deserted streets, shaking the mansion and sending the maids screaming, desperate to save falling bric-a-brac. The mayor took Viola into his arms, and then turned to the little gathering with a heavy sigh. "And, nae, I fear it is time."

⚬⚬⚭⚬

Charles and Simon carefully hoisted the cloth-covered portrait into the center of the crowded kitchen cart. Archie and the maids struggled to keep the upended painting from tipping sideways in the churning, ash-filled winds. As fast as he could flick away the burning cinders, more landed, leaving tiny burn marks upon the linen cloth. Yet another set of explosions rocked the cart, jarring their already frayed nerves. Jane shrieked and hid her head in her hands. Cecil grabbed the rails for balance as the cart settled.

"Mind your step, sweeting," cautioned Cecil as he handed a stoic Viola into the bay with the staff, and then looked to Catherine, Simon and Charles still standing on the lane. "Next?"

Simon was the first to speak. "I'm afraid I must return to the hospital."

"Nonsense, my boy!" cried Cecil. "You've not slept in days!"

Simon smiled, ruefully. "I fear I have nowhere to lay my head at the moment."

Viola stood in the cart and set her hands to the railings. "You are family now, Simon" She gestured toward the mansion. "Bealeton House is as much your home as it is ours…"

The ground shook with another mighty explosion that shot sparks and flames hundreds of feet into the sky on the east side of the park. Bricks fell off the side of the mansion, shattering dully as they hit the earth below. Viola grabbed onto the mayor for balance. "…for as long as it stands," she added, with a wry glance toward the detritus that began to shower down the sides of the mansion.

"And I intend to remain with Simon," said Catherine, taking his arm.

At that, Jane gathered her skirts, and began to climb down from the cart. She looked wide-eyed and nervous, but determined. "I..I'll stay with ye, Milady," she said, unconvincingly, glancing at the blood-red sky. She was clearly terrified as she stood in the dirt path, her skirts quivering as she shook from head to toe.

"Nae, Jane," said Gussie. "Eliza'll be needin' yer help at the Abbey."

Jane gasped as though she had just won a prize. "Oh, thank ye ever so much, Gussie," she breathed. She narrowed her eyes at the older woman. "Aye'n yer sure, nae?" Without waiting for an answer, Jane quickly climbed back up to the cart and settled herself on the bench. "'Tis me father that'll be needin' me at home, like as not," she murmured to anyone listening.

Viola turned toward Catherine as though she wished to mount a protest. Cecil placed a cautionary hand upon her knee. Viola glanced at him sharply, and then sighed. "As much as I would wish for you to be well away at the Abbey, your place is with your husband—as mine is with Cecil." She pointed directly at Simon. "Keep her safe, young man." She turned to Charles, standing to the side, firmly in lockstep with his sister. Viola placed her hands upon her hips. "And you... I suppose you intend to stay as well?"

"Yes, Aunt," he ventured, a bright red flush rising at his newfound independence. He lifted his chin. "I intend to ride to the east to find the Duke and vouchsafe that the firebreak holds. If not, I shall raise the alarm here."

Gussie stood and sighed. "Aye'n I will stay back as well. I 'spect these three'll be needin' a good meal or so in the comin' days." Archie handed her down from the cart. "Eliza n' Annie can cook fer ye at the Abbey 'till I return."

"I shall send the cart back loaded with provisions from the larder in the morning," said Cecil. "Fresh horses from the stables and the Abbey's carriage, as well, as I daresay it might be some time before a new one can be procured."

Archie stood and grabbed their bag from the bay of the cart. He threw it to the ground, and then disembarked himself, tipping his cap to Viola. "Mum." He turned and stood, placing his arm firmly around Gussie's shoulders. "Wells was more than enough. I'll not be separated from ye again, m'love," he whispered, squeezing her tight. Gussie leaned her head against his shoulder and wiped a tear from her eye.

Viola looked down to the five determined faces standing on the lane, illuminated by the fiery glow from the east and cocked an eyebrow. With one last glance toward her beloved mansion, Viola turned away and took a seat on the bench. She knew when she had been bested. "Very well, then." She lifted her chin. "Mr. Fitch!" she commanded, throwing her cloak over her shoulders. "Drive on."

CHAPTER SEVENTEEN

5 September 1666

She knelt down next to him in the candlelight's pale glow, gently washing the ashes from his skin with a fragrant soap made from soft, golden tallow and lye. With every stroke of the cloth, the lamentable memories of Dorcas and the untold others that Simon could not help began to slowly fade from his troubled thoughts. Her gentle hands spread the lather across his arms and chest, her tender ministrations calming his aching soul. Warmed on the fire and brought in buckets to the small wash chamber's half-barrel wood bath, the fresh hyssop-scented water felt good upon his burnt flesh. Catherine rinsed away the fire's filthy residue with gentle strokes of a cloth. Simon leaned back and closed his eyes, nearly giving into the sleep that threatened.

A slight rustle of fabric grazed his forehead. He opened his eyes. Catherine stood over him in a thin, silken nightshift that clung to every exquisite curve of her body, the wreath of ivory roses still crowning her copper curls. He could hear the nearby gun powder explosions. He felt the massive concussions shaking the house. It didn't matter. Nothing mattered, but her. Simon rose from the bath. The water streamed in rivulets down his thewy, muscular frame and fell back into the tub. He carefully removed the crown of roses, and then untied the laces binding her nightshift, slowly lifting the shift high above her head. He dropped the gown to the floor in a graceless heap and stared, mesmerized by the taut, elegant figure standing before him. His knees buckled at the sight of her soft smile. He sank back into the tub. Her ivory skin glowed in the candlelight. Tears dampened his cheeks, so choked with emotion was he by the miracle that she had consented to be his wife. Her delicate beauty dazzled Simon as she stood by the bath, soapy cloth in hand. She made no attempt to cover herself as she dropped the cloth into the water, then leaned over the wooden barrel staves and kissed the top of his head. He closed his eyes, relishing the soft touch of her lips. He was excited beyond measure. She kissed the tip of his nose and his cheeks, and then, her lips tenderly grazed his. Every single nerve ending tingled as he inhaled the sweet fragrance of orange blossom and wild thyme in the curls that fell upon his skin. He gazed at her in wonderment. Then, Simon rose once more. He stepped from the bath and swung her high into his arms. Unable to contain himself any longer, Simon kissed her lips, and then carried his bride straight up three flights of stairs to their chamber, setting the latch firmly behind them.

"Please, sir," cried a small voice, intruding into the tender thoughts of Catherine lying next to him, her soft skin pressing against his own in her sleep. He had lain awake for as long as possible, not daring to move lest it had all been a dream.

"Please, sir, help me find me mum!"

Disoriented, Simon looked down to see a little girl standing before him, clutching his tunics. He had not been paying attention. He stepped back and lifted his eyes, gazing across the grounds of St. Bartholomew's in astonishment. Four days after the fire began, the winds had at last died down and the firebreaks to the west had miraculously held, though a nauseating, acrid stench lingered thick above the vast, smoking ashes of what was once the great city of London. Simon stood at the entrance, shocked to see that hundreds of refugees with nowhere else to live now crowded the hospital grounds, taking shelter in ragged, makeshift tents. He looked down once more." Help me find me mum!" she screamed again, pulling desperately on his clothing. "Me mum!" she sobbed.

A man ran across the grassy forecourt and pulled the little girl away. He swung her up into his arms. "Beggin' yer pardon, sir, y'see's, she's 'ad quite a shock." He placed the little girl's head on his shoulder and bounced softly to calm her. "'Tis all right, nae. Shhhhh, Masie, 'tis all right." He leaned toward Simon. "She's so young, sir," he said, choking back the tears. "I canna tell her." The man held the crying girl close, wrapping her tight in his arms. Simon stared, helpless, as father and daughter walked back toward the silent, traumatized crowd.

Shaken by the encounter, Simon turned and took hold of the thick, iron door latch, more than apprehensive as to the reception he would receive from Father Hardwicke this day. He knew he had left the hospital when the needs had been dire. He had slipped out like a thief in the night, leaving the scores of injured and burned to the others who were surely exhausted and stretched to the limit without his help. The guilt was near unbearable. *Aye, surely Father Hardwicke will understand that Catherine had been injured.* He walked past the choked registration desk. The registrar was still there, sorting the horribly injured from the shocked and hysterical. The fat little man looked up and scowled at Simon, jerking his head toward the administration offices with an incomprehensible sneer.

His bravado shrinking, Simon walked into the administrator's building and faced the door. He raised his hand, and then knocked softly, waiting for the administrator's thin, reedy voice to bade him admittance. He was surprised when a deep voice came from within.

"Enter."

Simon put his thumb on the latch and pushed down. The door was stuck. He set his shoulder to the planks and shoved. The door gave way, swinging wide. He stumbled into the dim chamber, his eyes widening in surprise at the sight of Dr. Godfrey Palgrave sitting behind the administrator's desk as he caught his balance. The old man, looking for all the world as though he belonged there, drew a heavy sigh as he waited for Simon to compose himself. The silence was unbearable.

"Two days, McKensie," the old physician finally barked.

Simon glanced away, for the physician's stringy, greasy hair, his dirty fingernails and his bloodstained, filthy tunics made his stomach lurch. He mustered a modicum of formality. "Aye, sir. There was a carriage accident. My betrothed was injured, and Sister Rosamond bade me…"

"I have no interest in your personal affairs, McKensie!" shouted Dr. Palgrave, interrupting any attempts to an explanation.

Simon fell silent. *Dear God, how he despised this man.* "Father Hardwicke knew of my absence…"

Dr. Palgrave cut him off. "Father Hardwicke lies this hour in a profoundly lethargic state, neither able to speak nor comprehend a word spoken."

"I beg your pardon?"

"Aye. Beaten nearly to death for a trinket of gold," he spat in disgust. He stared at Simon. "Whether he lives or dies is nae entirely up to the will of God."

Shocked, Simon took a moment to comprehend the words. *Father Hardwicke beaten? Profoundly lethargic?* His thoughts immediately turned to the Lord Mayor. "He does not know," Simon murmured aloud.

"What?" the physician barked.

"His brother, the Lord Mayor of Wells escaped the fires and returned to Stockbridge. He does not know of Father Hardwicke's injuries."

Dr. Palgrave twisted his thin lips into a snarl. "His brother is of no interest to me, either. You may send word on your own time. What does interest me, however, is that as senior physician, I am now Head Administrator of this hospital until such time as Father Hardwicke recovers. Which could well be months—*if* at all." He fixed Simon with a distorted grimace, baring yellowing teeth that were blackened at the gum line. Several were missing altogether. Simon fought the urge to be sick. "And as such, that God-forsaken, sacrilegious dissectory of yours has at this hour been dismantled," Dr. Palgrave continued, drawing the 's' out much like the hissing of a snake, "for I believe the practice sheer heresy, not to mention an abominable affront to God, himself. 'Tis incomprehensible that Father Hardwicke would allow such experimentation."

Were he not stunned beyond comprehension, Simon would have savored the paradox of a forward thinking, scientifically curious *priest* who's own religious views allowed for medical experimentation and research, set against this barbarous, filthy, superstitious and backward-thinking cretin spouting the will of God in Father Hardwicke's stead. But he was not thinking straight. "No!" cried Simon, incredulous at the swiftly turning events. He rose to his feet, grasping for any straw. "You cannot do that! I've not nearly research enough—I need more time, far more experimentation!"

"I can." Dr. Palgrave unlaced his fingers and leaned across the desk. His voice dropped to a dangerous octave. "And I have." He banged his hands on the wood. "If I could, I would discharge you of your duties at St. Bartholomew's altogether." Palgrave paused a moment and stared with utter contempt at this brash, intelligent and, in his singular estimation, woefully undisciplined physician standing before him. He exhaled. "However, since we are overwhelmed from the fire and are likely to remain so as the refugee situation worsens, you may complete the final two months of your residency—*at your own expense.* If, at the turn of the calendar year, Father Hardwicke has not recovered, your continued employment will be evaluated. Until then, you may oversee only the bonesetters, or treat only the fevers. I do not care which."

Simon stared in astonishment that this man, *nae, this barbarian,* who, along with Dr. Clarke, had opposed every single idea, every single piece of research and knowledge, every last theory Simon had advanced throughout his years of medical training was now in charge of his life.

"You may go."

With a curt wave of the old man's fingers, Simon looked as though his entire world had just collapsed. Dr. Palgrave watched with extraordinary satisfaction as Simon quietly left the chamber, then rose and walked into the anteroom adjacent to Hardwicke's office where he had seen several wooden containers stacked against a wall. The top slat of each container had been marked with the initials S. M. A sudden curiosity, a spark of instantaneous connection fired in his scheming thoughts. *S. M.—Simon McKensie?* He closed the door to the anteroom, then with an iron letter opener from Father Hardwicke's desk, pried the top from one of the containers and began to rifle through the contents. *Blasphemous!* In his worst imaginings, he could think of no other word to describe the crude images he saw on the papers. *The human body split apart, much as one would gut a spring lamb.* Revulsion clutched at his stomach as he gazed with macabre fascination at the organs that had been drawn inside the gaping hole. He squinted carefully at the bottom of the first page. 'Mendicant No.' 1. *A beggar.* He lifted his head, thoughts swirling in his brain. *There were five such crates stacked one atop the other.* He looked closer at the drawing he held. Printed underneath the mendicant notation was a smudged signature. *S.M. Physick.* A noise from the hall startled him. He quickly stuffed the parchment back into the crate, replaced the lid and set an unopened crate on top. He waited until the noise died down, then stepped back and stared at the five wooden boxes, his febrile mind working hard to make sense of it all. He shook his head. *What has the fool done?*

❧

Catherine lay alone under a thick pile of quilts, and bit her thumbnail, savoring the delicious memory of the night before. *She was married.* She could scarcely believe it had happened, so unexpected and sudden was the ceremony, and yet, it had indeed taken place. She thought of Simon lying next to her in the dark, as he had once before on a soft, moonlit night beneath a gnarled oak tree. The night her father died. *The night she gave the broken pieces of her heart to the man she loved beyond measure.*

Catherine rolled over and buried her face in the goose down pillow next to hers, inhaling deeply of the rugged, masculine scent left behind on the smooth linen coverings.

He had awakened her in the quiet of the early morning, pressing his lips, warm and tender, into the gentle curve of her back, as if to memorize completely the soft swells, the gentle arcs and delicate clefts of her body. Gathering her into the strong, muscular curvature of his own body, they had lain together in the dark until two, at last, became one. His embrace was strong and sure. He held her with a tenderness that came from the quiet place deep in his heart. *He had loved her from the very moment they met.* Simon held her tight until exhaustion overtook them both. They lay wrapped in each other's arms until a lone rooster on the street outside crowed at dawn. He lay beside her, watching until she stirred. She smiled and murmured his name, then snuggled deeper into the pillow and drifted off once more. Reluctantly rising, Simon kissed her forehead, then quietly slipped out to the hospital, leaving a trace of lemon balm in the air behind him.

Yawning, a sleepy Catherine reached for the watchcase on the table beside the bed. She turned it over to read the inscription once more. *4 September 1666.* She held the watch to her chest and reveled in the silence. *The silence!* With a start, she realized that she had not heard or felt an explosion in hours. *The firebreaks have held!* She threw the covers back and ran to the window, pulling the curtains aside. Through the smoke-streaked panes, she could see the autumn leaves hanging still on the London plane tree fronting the mansion. The winds had died down overnight and the smoke in the air was beginning to settle in the West End. She looked across the park toward the city. Fallow, stagnant clouds of ash hung heavy over the smoking ruins of London, as thick and ominous as the day the fire began. Unflinching tears spilled down her cheeks. *What of the people? What's to become of them?* She wiped her cheeks and stared at the thick, smoking remains. *It was all so terribly heartbreaking.* She turned away, unable to look upon the disaster any longer. She sighed, briefly wondering where Jane was with her morning toilette. A sudden pang of guilt pierced her conscience like the tip of a needle. She clutched the velvet window hangings and saw, in her mind's eye, the accusing look on the old man's face as he had bumped into the carriage. *He was right.* She was indeed privileged, and never more so than this very morning. *She still had a home.*

Gussie knocked softly on the door, and then entered quietly carrying a tray. Seeing Catherine awake at the window, she smiled and set the tray on a table at the side of the bed. "Good morning t' ye's…" she paused and smiled, "…Lady McKensie." Catherine dropped the curtains and ran into the stout cook's outstretched arms. "Congratulations, my lamb, Archie'n me, why we couldn't be more cock-a-hoop for ye's both. We wish you and the good doctor many years of happiness together."

An inexplicable melancholy seemed to settle over Catherine. "Oh, Gussie, I feel as though I've no right to happiness, when so many are this day suffering such unbearable loss."

In the quiet of the early morning hour, neither woman spoke for a moment. The desolation outside the paned windows seemed so very far away. A ceiling truss cracked from the unsettling explosions the night before as Gussie took Catherine's face into her capable old hands. The older woman looked into the earnest eyes of the sweet girl she'd helped raise like she was her very own. "Ah, m'lassie, the good Lord didna' bless Archie n' me with wee ones, but you and Charlesie are me own lambkins all the same, y'are. An' ye've as much right to yer own happiness, just the same as anybody else." Gussie set hands upon Catherine's shoulders and spoke with determination. "I'll not allow ye to sacrifice yer joy this mornin' on account'a the fire." She leaned in, close. "'Tis nobody's fault, and 'tis certainly no fault of yer own. Remember that, my love."

Catherine's eyes filled with tears, yet again. "What would I do without you, Gussie?"

Gussie wiped the tears from Catherine's face with the hem of her apron. "Ah, get on with ye, lassie," she smiled and threw the window hangings wide, flooding the room with a strange yellow light. "Nae, Archie's heating water for the bath. I thought ye's might like a good soak..." She poured the tea and, crossing the warm, feminine chamber, handed the cup to Catherine, "...but perhaps ye might like a few more winks, instead?"

"No, Gussie, no more sleep. A bath would be lovely, indeed."

Gussie handed Catherine a robe from the armoire that stood next to the doorway. "Er'e ye be," she said, helping Catherine into the green velvet dressing gown. "And the rest of yer day? What 'ave ye and Simon planned?"

"Simon left for the hospital early this morning, and I don't know exactly when he will return..." Catherine hesitated a moment, "...however, as soon as the horses and carts return from the Abbey, I believe I should like to visit Moorfield's Park."

"Moorfield's Park? Whatever for?" asked Gussie, plumping the pillows.

Catherine stared through the window to the ash and detritus that lay thick upon the deserted thoroughfare, and then turned to Gussie, thoughtfully. "I...I am not entirely sure. Charles said last night that the refugees have gathered there." She bit her fingernail, musing. "Perhaps I can offer help somehow. I do not really know—it just seems that perhaps I should try."

"The cookery's cart'll likely be loaded with stock from the Abbey larder," said Gussie. "I s'pose Archie n' me ken' lend a hand." She narrowed her gaze at Catherine. "Yer very much like yer father, indeed," she smiled, her hooded eyes softening at the memory of the kind and generous Abbott family patriarch. "'E were always tryin' to help this one or that."

Catherine took another sip of tea in the quiet chamber, and then set the cup to the tray. "There was a moment before the accident, Gussie."

Gussie tugged the bedclothes into place with a snap. "Aye?"

"An old man willfully collided with the carriage as we were trapped in the escaping crowds. When I looked through the glass, he was standing there in the lane, staring at me. T'was but a fleeting moment, but in that moment, Gussie, I saw something in his eyes." She looked to the old cook, her brows furrowed in concern. "I confess it troubled me greatly."

"What was it, lass?"

"I don't know," her voice trailed off as she relived the unsettling encounter in her mind's eye. "A silent reproach, perhaps? A condemnation? It was as though he knew me. Perhaps not me in particular, but someone like me. I…I felt an enormous guilt as though I had been judged, Gussie. Judged and found wanting."

Gussie smiled softly. "And so…to Moorfield's."

Catherine nodded, determination setting in. "Yes. To Moorfield's."

CHAPTER EIGHTEEN

"UNEASY LIES THE HEAD THAT WEARS THE CROWN"
~ WILLIAM SHAKESPEARE

River Thames
London, England
6 September 1667

Red-painted oars pulled rhythmically into the calm waters of the Thames, each stroke splashing water droplets that sparkled in the glare of the rising sun. Rounding a bend in the river, King Charles II arose from his throne at the rear and raised his fist. At once, the eight sailors to a man, set the oars across their knees and stared forward, as the shallop bobbed on the ash-covered water. He walked forward and stared, incredulous, at the vast, smoldering ruins of what was but five short days ago the magnificent city of London.

If asked, he would be incapable of putting into words the desolation, the rage, and the utter helplessness he felt so very deep in his soul at the melancholy sight. It is gone, he thought sadly, as he stared at the city from his vantage point on the debris-choked river. *It is all gone.* He was overwhelmed by the enormity of it all. From the walls of the West End to the Tower of London in the east, blackened timbers of buildings both opulent and humble lay in a twisted, chaotic jumble. Though the fires were largely extinguished, lamentable plumes of smoke rose from nearly every quarter. The familiar, comforting spires of St. Paul's Cathedral on Ludgate Hill had burned to the ground, its lead roof still molten, seeping red-hot. King Henry VIII's favorite retreat, the rambling, riverfront Bridewell Palace lay in ruin, its majestic brick ramparts collapsing into a smoking pile. Even the vast, open-air, four-storied trading piazza of the Royal Exchange lay in smoldering ruin. *It was all in ruins.*

He felt weak in direful contemplation of the enormous financial losses. The cost to rebuild would be staggering. Were it not for the oarsmen, he would have wept, such was the desolation, the sickening, roiling desolation that befell him at the sight of his city. He sagged unceremoniously to a storage box at the bow and set his head to his hands. Awake for nearly five days he was exhausted in the extreme, sickened by the knowledge that the worst days, weeks, years, even, lay ahead. *He was the loneliest man in the world.* Something bumped softly into the side of the bow, jostling him from his woes. He looked over the railing to see a young girl of about ten, dressed in a pink gown, floating dead in the river. *He could take no more.* He turned to the head oarsman with tears in his eyes.

"Away."

CHAPTER NINETEEN

"WE ARE BECOME LIKE WORMS, THAT ONLY LIVE IN THE
DULL EARTH OF IGNORANCE, WINDING OURSELVES
SOMETIMES OUT BY THE HELP OF SOME REFRESHING
RAIN OF GOOD EDUCATION, WHICH SELDOM IS GIVEN
US, FOR WE ARE KEPT LIKE BIRDS IN CAGES."
~LADY MARGARET CAVENDISH

Bealeton House
St. James Parish, London
26 October 1666

MaryPryde gripped the rough, splintered side rail of the horse cart and stared wide-eyed, at the stately brick mansion that seemed to rise to the very heavens above. She was astonished that one family lived in such elegant splendor. Her knees began to shake.

"Bealeton House," barked the driver, crowding into her panicked thoughts. He glanced back at his motionless passenger and sighed. "We've arrived, Miss," he said, more kindly.

MaryPryde jerked her head toward the driver and nodded. "Aye." She pulled a small silver coin from the pocket of her skirts, and held it toward the gruff man with trembling hands.

He looked her over from head to toe, and sighed. "Nae, Miss. Ye looks as if ye needs it more." He waved her down from the cart. "Off with ye. Off with ye, a'fore I change me mind."

MaryPryde quickly pocketed the coin. "Oh, thank ye, sir," she breathed, climbing down to the elegant, tree-lined courtyard. "I'm grateful to ye." The driver clicked his teeth and the rickety cart trundled away.

She examined the card in her hand once more and then looked up to compare the address to the brass plaque affixed to one of the two formidable pillars fronting the mansion. *'Tis Bealeton House, indeed.* She took a deep breath, tightened the grip on the handle of her bag and climbed the steps to the immaculate, white-painted front door. She took hold of the iron knocker and clunked it dully against the back plate. The flittering butterflies in her stomach grew stronger. Within moments, the door opened.

"Yes, Miss?" asked a plump woman wearing an apron and a kind smile.

MaryPryde held out the calling card that Catherine had slipped into the book. "Is…is Lady Abbott at home?" MaryPryde flinched in her boots, resisting a desperate urge to turn tail and run.

"She is out, Miss." Gussie reached for the card and looked closely at the print. "Is she expectin' ye?"

MaryPryde looked down to the ground. "Nae." MaryPryde dipped in a slight curtsey. "Beggin' yer pardon, mum, for the intrusion." She retrieved the card, and then turned, slipping it back into her pocket of her skirt. She started down the steps toward the street.

"If I may, Miss…" Gussie called out after her.

MaryPryde turned back, a wary flash of fear in her eyes. "Aye?"

"D'yes have a name?"

MaryPryde thought fast. Flynt was surely dead in the fire. No one but Lady McKensie knew she had been married but two days. *Should she use Pollard, or the name she was born with?* She lifted her chin. "Beckwith, mum," she said. "MaryPryde Beckwith."

"Aye, Miss Beckwith. And how did ye's happen to come by th' card?"

"Lady Abbott gave it to me, she did. At the hospital. Before the fire." MaryPryde reached into her bag and proffered Simon's medical book "She put it in this book," protested MaryPryde.

Gussie took a closer look at the book. "Why tha' belongs to Doctor McKensie."

"I didna' pinch it," MaryPryde whispered, tears welling in her eyes. "I…I only wanted to give it back."

"Ah, Miss, I did'na' say ye did," sighed Gussie, stepping out into the daylight. She wiped her hands on her apron, and then set hand to forehead, squinting in the sun. "She's called Lady McKensie, nae," she said, kindly.

"I dinna' know, mum. I only met her the once. At the hospital before the fire, like I said." She looked away, embarrassed. "I…I was hurt, an' she took care of me."

Gussie cocked her head, contemplating. There was something in the girl's humble manner, in her dignified bearing that belied her young years, yet she could not place her finger on the perplexity. "Are ye on the mend, then?" Gussie suddenly twigged onto it. *The girl was alone on the step.* Gussie could not hold her tongue. "Yer family takin' good care of ye?"

"Aye. T'was nothing."

"Huumph," said Gussie, crossing her arms.

MaryPryde knew Gussie would find her response wanting. She glanced to the street, quickly taking the measure of the long walk back to Moorfield's Park where she had taken refuge with thousands of others escaping the fires after she ran from Flynt Pollard. She did not exactly know whether the man was alive or dead. *But, she knew she was tired.* Tired of being hungry. Tired of sleeping curled under a bush, of waking in fear at every footstep in the night. Tired of being scared and penniless. On this day, MaryPryde awoke, collected her wits and the few coins she had earned from repairing the worn clothes of the refugees, and with one single purpose mind, went searching for Lady Catherine Abbott. *She needed a job.* "I have no family. I…I have no home."

"Where d'yes lay yer head, girl?"

She hesitated. "Since the fire, I've been sleeping in Moorfield's Park."

Gussie looked the young woman over, from the top of her neatly plaited hair to the toes of her worn, but clean, lace-up boots. She crossed her arms over her ample bosom, and gave a small harrumph. "Ye look hungry."

"Nae, mum," MaryPryde said softly. She looked to the ground, embarrassed once again.

"Nonsense. Yer gown hangs off yer bones," Gussie said, emphatically. "Come inside, lass. I'll cook you up a right, proper meal."

MaryPryde stood, wavering, unsure as to what to do.

Gussie cocked an eyebrow. "Come along, girl," she said, brooking no nonsense.

MaryPryde followed Gussie and stepped into the cool, darkened mansion. Once inside, her eyes adjusted to the dim light. She stopped short and gazed slack-jawed at the spacious entrance hall, dazzled by the gleaming marble flooring, the massive, hand carved wooden bannister up to the portrait gallery, and the sparkling glass-dropped candelabras lining the ivory-colored plastered walls. *And the silence.* T'was the kind of elegant silence that betokened great wealth. *Not once in her simple imaginings had she er'e dared to dream of such magnificence.* She closed her eyes and inhaled the sweet scent of beeswax, letting her thoughts wander. And wander, they did. *She was smiling. Dressed in an elegant, golden green gown that matched her eyes, she gracefully swept down the marble stairs to an extravagant ballroom filled with dancing, music and laughter.* A sudden clattering of feet on the wooden floor of the gallery that rimmed the entrance hall above cut short her daydream.

"Gussie!" shouted an urgent voice.

MaryPryde looked up sharply toward a tousled mop of red hair that poked over the balcony.

"Aye, Milord?"

"Would you ask Archie to please saddle Ganymeade?" He waved a copy of the London Gazette. "Robert Hubert is to be hanged at Tyburn today." He tossed the broadsheet down to her from the balcony.

"Milord!" exclaimed Gussie, as she deftly caught the fluttering paper. She rolled it up and shook it up at him. "I dinna' wish to see this enquirin' rag!" She glanced down to the blaring headline on Hubert. "Aye, the way they trumpet the worst of humanity, whether it's the God's truth or not," she groused. "Why, the very idea, ruinin' lives merely for the coin of it." She shoved the newspaper into her apron pocket, and then looked from Charles to MaryPryde. "We 'ave a guest, Milord."

Charles followed her glance, surprised to see a young woman standing in the entrance hall. He descended the staircase, winding his cravat tightly about his neck. A deep blue, wool jacket dangled unceremoniously over the crook of his arm. "I beg your pardon, Miss! I did not realize we had a visitor," he smiled, bowing slightly. "Please allow me to introduce myself. I am Charles Abbott." Momentarily rendered mute by the flurry of activity, MaryPryde stood fast, staring at the grinning, ginger-haired young man. "And you are…?" he asked, gently.

"MaryPryde, sir," she murmured, bowing her head.

"Robert Hubert, Milord?" Gussie mused aloud. "The name's familiar."

Charles turned his attention back to Gussie. "'Tis the French man who confessed to setting the fire."

"Ah, yes, the French rapscallion. He confessed to it, right as rain."

"After spending a week in White Lion prison, he has been tried, found guilty, and is to be hanged today," he said, tipping his head to MaryPryde. "Begging your pardon again, Miss."

MaryPryde nodded, fascinated by the thought of a hanging.

"'Tis confusing though, Gussie, for Hubert has confessed to throwing the fireball a full two days *after* the fire started, yet he claims full responsibility," said Charles, pacing, working to comprehend the whole of it. "How can it possibly be that despite the obvious incompatibility of the testimony—and I have heard it said that he may well be deprived of reason—they intend to proceed with the public execution." He turned back and paced , logically working through the argument. "I can see that as a Frenchman, and therefore most likely a papist, there is much anger amongst Londoners toward the poor wretch—and yet, surely the judge would not allow the angry sentiment of our citizens to dictate the rule of law by proceeding with the hanging if he were not fully in command of his wits…"

Charles turned back to see Gussie and MaryPryde staring at him, completely bewildered. He instantly fell silent, chagrined once more. "My apologies for prattling on, please forgive me once more, Miss." He turned to Gussie with a soft smile. "There is no need to disturb Archie, I shall attend to the horse myself." He walked out the front door, and then suddenly ducked back inside, his manners returning. "Good day to you, Miss."

MaryPryde blushed and bowed her head.

Gussie saw the girl's reddening cheeks and turned her head slightly to conceal a smile. She cleared her throat.

Gussie set her hands to her ample hips and cocked an eyebrow at the gangly young girl. "I don't reckon ye can cook, can ye?"

MaryPryde knew an opportunity when it came along. She seized upon the moment. "Aye, I can, mum. I can, indeed! I can sew as well, an' I can clean, an…an' bake, an'… "

"All right, Miss," said Gussie, raising her hands in mock surrender. She smiled once more. "I su'pos'e ye ought t' follow me, then," Gussie said, briskly composing herself as she led the girl to the belowstairs cookery.

❧

Catherine was not alone in her guilt. She had traveled to Moorfield's Park nearly every day for weeks, as had so many other fortunate souls from the West End whose homes and lives had been spared in the last, desperate effort to save Whitehall Palace. Though the hospital to the north and Bealeton House and the palace to the west lay outside the London wall, both Catherine and Simon had traveled into the city proper to witness for themselves the sheer immensity of the destruction. Both were shaken, as were all who beheld the devastated city, to see that nearly every structure lay burnt and destroyed in smoldering ash. Contemplating the ruined lives and property left an ache so deep that in both gratitude and humbling guilt, all manner of carts and carriages, from the modest to the elegant, lined the edges of Moorfield's Park with offerings of food, clothes, blankets and wood for both cooking and warmth, for the cold of winter was fast approaching and the refugees were desperate. Whatever could be spared was generously given by those who had to those who had not.

Rocking gently in the bay of the cookery's horse cart as Fitch guided the horses to the edge of the park, Catherine gazed out at the vast greensward now bursting with thousands of refugees as far as one could see and sighed at the thought that had been troubling her since the carriage accident. *What's to become of them?* She tipped her head back and felt the soft October sun shining warm upon her face. The acrid scent of burnt oil and iron smelt from the ravaged shipping warehouses still lingered in the air, fouling the crisp autumn scent of fallen leaves. Shouts of laughter from a scrappy ring of boys playing swords with sticks caught her attention. She smiled, relishing their exuberance.

"Ah, the gladsome hearts of children, eh' Milady?" laughed Fitch, watching the horseplay as he readied the wooden barrels of water and ladles. "'Tis their very good fortune to live in youthful ignorance."

"Yes, Mr. Fitch, they look happy, indeed," she smiled. She rose and began to untie the strings of ten rough borel-lap cloth bags full of bread for the line of refugees that would soon form.

A young woman wearing an over-large men's cloak made her way up to the cart. The woman clung tightly to a dark-haired little girl whose shoulders were covered by a tattered quilt. Though the woman stood barefoot in the grass, the little girl had strips of cloth tied around her tiny feet to protect them from the detritus of camp living that was now strewn across the park. Catherine handed down the first of the sweet, fragrant bread loaves.

A lone chicken clucked nearby, pecking uselessly at the dirt for scraps of food. The little girl wrenched her hand away and ran to chase the bird. The outraged chicken squawked in loud protest and skittered away as the girl grabbed hold of its flapping wings. She sank to the ground and began to cry. The mother quickly scooped the little girl up into her arms and soothed her with a torn piece of the bread. "Thank ye Miss," whispered the mother as she nodded, her eyes downcast and troubled. Though she was yet young, her sallow, worn face belayed the worries and cares of those still taking shelter in the park these many weeks after the fire. She looked aged far beyond her years. Catherine watched with tears in her eyes as the pair waded back into the makeshift refugee village cluttered with ragged tents, cook fires and miserable human offal. Catherine wiped her eyes and turned her attention back to the long line that had formed, handing down another loaf to the next man in line.

"Thank you, indeed," murmured the gentleman. He reached up to take the bread in hand, and then, straightening the lapel of his filthy, but costly waistcoat with a proper tug, smiled a sad smile before melting back into the crowd. She did not know him, but she *knew* him. *She had socialized with, danced with, and feasted with so many just like this man and his family.* Though clearly from considerable means, just as the plague had done the year before, the fire had affected the lives of everyone in ways they could never have expected. The fire had reduced not only this dignified man, but all manner of London society's unfortunate souls to beggars. *Great wealth or crushing poverty made not a jot of difference when everything one had was gone.* The sprawling, filthy park that lay before her was proof enough of that. A wave of sadness washed over her at the sight of it. She handed down yet another loaf of bread.

The king himself had made several visits to the vast encampment urging the dispossessed to move on from the park, indeed to leave London altogether, but many had nowhere to go. Others simply refused. Rough-hewn shelters had begun to appear under the tree-studded acreage, giving rise to communal bonds of necessity. Over these last weeks, Catherine watched as those who could sew began to encamp next to those who would wash. Those who could cook drew the company of those who could chop wood and keep the fires lit. Slowly, a hint of order was beginning to emerge from the unending chaos. *Some may never leave.* Catherine slowly folded the last empty, coarse borel-lap bag and set it on the bench with the rest. She had handed down thirty loaves of bread.

With no other use for her time since Simon's dissectory had been dismantled, she and Gussie had worked together to bake ten loaves of bread each day while Simon was at the hospital. The rest of the loaves were ordered on the Bealeton accounts from Povey's Baker's, Ltd. in his West End shop near the mansion. Though it had been a quiet, settled time with Simon, and she had treasured every moment of her new marriage, a growing restlessness had begun to gnaw at her when he was absent. The fire had upended her life as much as it had nearly everyone in London. *Strange that she had once escaped a marriage of privilege and idleness to now feel so terribly unsettled by the guilt of both privilege and idleness.* At times, she felt as though she were a caged animal, pacing about at all hours while Simon slept, frustrated by an overwhelming sense of something odd, yet oddly definable. *A lack of purpose. A lack of accomplishment.* Though she dare not give voice to it, she knew Simon felt it, too, for the lack of authority at the hospital and his sheer frustration with Dr. Palgrave had been causing Simon vexations, as well.

She had tried to make herself useful. She had worked hard to put the house back to rights, though workmen to repair the cracked plaster were in high demand in the city and repairs to the damage would have to wait. With Jane writing that she had returned to her father's farm, and the rest of the Abbey staff staying in Stockbridge, she and Simon rattled around the house with Charles, Gussie and Archie. She found that she rather liked her newfound privacy. She enjoyed dressing herself, arranging her own hair into a simple knot. She never had taken pleasure in being waited upon, although Gussie and Archie certainly could use an extra set of hands while Charles waited for a navigational assignment on another supply ship to the colonies. Aunt Viola had sent word that she would stay in the country until the London she once knew arose from the smoldering ashes. Though she knew her aunt was prone to exaggeration and would soon return, Catherine looked over the treetops toward the faint smoke still hovering over the burned-out city. *It may take years before London rises again,* thought Catherine, sadly.

Distant hoof beats clopping dully in the lane behind her began to grow louder. Catherine looked back to witness a fashionable black carriage approaching the park. Gravel crunched as the elegant, brass-trimmed coach rolled slowly to a stop next to the cart. The coach's driver pulled back on the reins and secured them to the handbrake. He threw several bundles of clothing down to the grass, and then dismounted, himself. Setting a wooden footstool on the ground, the uniformed driver opened the carriage door. A vast, plumed hat emerged first. Catherine watched in fascination as a woman stepped from the carriage, dressed in an elaborate costume of black and purple taffeta silk. A massive ruffle adorned the collar, matched only by the singular ruffled train falling from the coach as the woman stepped down. Catherine furrowed her brow in momentary confusion. *She had seen this woman before.* She had seen her that day in the publishing house. *'Tis Lady Margaret Cavendish!* The spectacularly attired woman turned to her. She narrowed her eyes in deep thought, and then suddenly smiled softly. "I know you," she said in her quiet, whispery voice. "Butterflies."

CHAPTER TWENTY

Bealeton House
St. James Parish, London
27 October 1666
3:00am

Fyrst Sleep. A right peculiar name fer it, groused Gussie to herself, as she lay wide-awake in her simple bedchamber belowstairs listening once again to the cookery's workclock chime thrice. She rolled over and sighed. 'Tis an interminable mid-life vexation, to be sure. It was a commonly enough prescribed remedy that one should rise in the night for an hour or two of idle pursuit before settling back to a second sleep, but she was quite sure that those doing the prescribing had no earthly notion of the irritation that wakenings in the night caused women of a certain age. That there was, in fact, a proper name for the awakenings made it only slightly more palatable. The knowledge that she was not alone in staring at the ceiling as the chimes rang one after the other in the night was only slightly less troubling, but no matter the lackbrained name for it, she desperately wished at two and fifty years that she could sleep the way she did when she was young. In truth, she felt as old as Methuselah in the bible stories taught to the wee ones in the nursery.

Archie snuffled and reached for her in the dark. The rope bed strained as she shifted her bulk to curl up in his old arms, letting her mind drift in the hopes that sleep would overtake once more. As she lay quiet, the beams above her snapped with soft footfalls, then creaks on the servant's stairs next to her chamber could be heard. *Someone was coming down.* Moving carefully so as to not awaken Archie, Gussie rose from the bedstead. She donned her heavy dressing gown and slipped into the narrow passageway, quietly latching the door behind her. She struck a flint to the thick candle sitting on the ledge outside her chamber just as Simon appeared at the bottom of the stairway. Startled, Gussie pushed her frizzled hair up into her nightcap in a hopeless attempt to straighten her appearance.

"Oh! Ye surprised me, Doctor McKensie! Thought it might be Catherine or Charles—they often come down fer a tuck in the night," she whispered.

"Please. Call me Simon," he said softly, as he took the candlestick from her to lead the way into the darkened cookery. "I…I only came down for a cup of tea, Mrs. Crawdor." He lifted the candlestick high, and stared in confusion at the enormous rack of gleaming copper pots and pans hanging from the low, barrel ceiling. "Can you tell me which pot I might use?"

Gussie struck the flint once more and lit a series of candles down the length of the planked servants table, illuminating the generous cookery with a soft light. "Nonsense, I'm happy to make the tea fer ye." She smiled and pointed to the long bench fronting the table. "Sit there, an' I'll have it for ye in a tick." She stoked the coals to flame, and then reached under a sideboard for a well-used copper pot. "And, if I'm t' call ye Simon, ye'd best call me Gussie," she said, filling the pot with water from the water barrel.

Simon took a seat, mesmerized by the flickering shadows cast by the candleflame upon the coved, brick ceiling arches. Gussie set the pot on an iron grate that hung by chains over the coals, then reached for two thick, crockery cups from a shelf above the wooden countertop. Setting them on the servant's table, she carefully measured a spoonful of loose tea leaves from a covered jar into the cups. She reached into another jar for a bit of hard candy sugar, then stopped and looked back at Simon. "Perhaps ye'd prefer a tot of brandy in yer tea, instead?" she asked with more than a hint of hope.

Simon smiled. "The sugar will be fine, Gussie."

Gussie looked slightly disappointed. "Aye," she said, sighing under her breath. She turned once more to the grate and, lifting the pot from the fire with a heavy cloth, poured the boiling water into a porcelain teapot that had been a gift to Lord Abbott from a visiting Dutch merchant. Several quiet minutes went by. "Yer unable to sleep?" she asked finally, pouring the fragrant brew into the two cups. She slid one toward Simon.

"Aye, I've a great deal on my mind."

Gussie cocked her head, setting the thick cloth to the wooden sideboard. "What's troublin' ye, if ye don't mind my askin'?" she said, brisk in her plainspoken ways.

Simon furrowed his brow, inexperienced as he was to unburdening his troubles on another soul. He played with the rim of the cup, then idly tapped the cup to the table and watched the tiny leaves float upwards from the bottom. The clock ticked, louder it seemed, with each passing second.

"Ye've made her very happy, Simon," ventured Gussie, breaking the quiet. "Happier than I've ever seen her before."

Simon looked up with sad, searching eyes. "Do you think so?" He looked into her wise, old face and suddenly felt an overwhelming sense of relief. His resolve crumbled as the weight of keeping his own counsel lifted from his soul. "She seems much troubled," he confessed. He fiddled with the rim of the cup once more. "I believe she misses our work in the dissectory as much as I do, and although I despise the position I now find myself in at the hospital, I can get through my days with the students. But there is a restlessness in her that I confess I feel responsible for, yet do not know how to remedy." The cup tipped in his fingers, spilling a bit of the tea onto the table. Distracted by his troubled thoughts, Simon seemed not to notice. "Perhaps if we returned to Stockbridge and the Abbey? Her soul seems to be at peace in the countryside."

Gussie considered the situation with her practical turn of

mind. "Perhaps Catherine might indeed be happier in the country—though why anyone would prefer the crickets to the excitement of the city is beyond my ken," murmured a bemused Gussie. After a moment, she set the cup firmly on the table and spoke directly. "I do not believe that anyone is responsible for the happiness of another, laddie." She idly swiped the pool of tea from the table with a calloused palm. "I have known—nae loved—Catherine since she was a wee lass, an' Simon, I have seen the rise and fall of her attentions to pursuits that make me old head spin in circles. I can tell ye that she and she alone will work her way through any restlessness she is wont to abide. Having ye by her side is all she needs."

Simon cleared his throat. He took a sip of tea to forestall the tears of relief that threatened to spill.

"Have ye spoken to her of yer concerns?" asked Gussie.

"Nae. She was long asleep by the time I came home from the hospital tonight. And even that is a great part of my concerns— my work separates us far more than I thought it might. I fear that I am forced to leave her alone during the days and now, at times, even the nights."

Gussie smiled. "Ah, laddie, she knew well of yer dedication and the hours yer profession required long before she agreed to marry ye. She's a woman grown, she is, an' my lambkins, well nigh' knows her own turn of mind." Gussie finished her tea and stood to clear. "Nae, Simon, " she pronounced with finality, "ye've no need to worry. I've seen this many a time before. Her interests and talents are many, an' she's nae one to settle upon one endeavor for long. Catherine's a resourceful and intelligent lass. She'll find herself a new pursuit, like as not."

Simon stood, relieved beyond words. "You've calmed my fears more than you can know, and I'm grateful to you, Gussie." He set his hand upon her arm, and then, for once, threw caution to the wind. He leaned down and gave her a tiny peck on the cheek.

Gussie gave a hearty grin, then picked up the cups for the washbucket and pushed him toward the door with her elbow. "Ahhh, get on with ye, nae. Back to bed, laddie—the sun will be a'risin' before ye know it."

"Good night, Gussie," he said, giving her a wink as he walked toward the dim passageway, feeling lighter than he had in weeks.

"Good night, lad," said Gussie. She leaned over the table and blew the candles out.

❦

Upstairs, in their third floor chamber, Simon crawled back under the still-warm bedcovers. Catherine felt the bedstead shake and murmured something he could not understand. She slid over, sleepily fitting herself into the curve of his body and sighed, content beyond measure. Simon wrapped his arms around her and knew Gussie was right, she would indeed find her way. He drifted off to a peaceful sleep holding her in his embrace. On the table by the bed, unseen in the dark, lay a hand-lettered envelope that had come by delivery that afternoon. Catherine's spirits had indeed lifted the moment it arrived. *An invitation to tea from Lady Margaret Cavendish.*

CHAPTER TWENTY-ONE

St. Bartholomew's Hospital
Smithfield Parish, London
29 October 1666

nough. Simon stood, arms crossed, to the side of a crude rope pallet in the great hall watching as a pale-faced, flustered first year student wrapped linen bindings around the broken leg of a workman who had tumbled from the scaffoldings that had begun to appear as the reconstruction of London commenced full-bore. Oswold Haggett tied the linen strips into a knot with shaking hands and then stood, accidentally dropping the leg to the floor. The unfortunate man's heel bounced off the wooden planks. He recoiled, screaming in agony. Simon rolled his eyes.

"Owww, sir!" cried the workman, looking to Simon with pleading eyes. "Me leg!" The workman grabbed at his thigh and raised his leg gingerly in the air. Tears dripped down his cheeks. "Me leg!" he bawled, "Me leg…"

Oswold cringed in wide-eyed horror. "My…my sincerest apologies, sir!" he whispered, slowly backing away from the patient. Though he looked frantically for an exit, there was no escaping the sharp eyes of Simon McKensie.

For two interminable months, Simon had gritted his teeth working with the bonesetters, the most junior of medical students that populated the hospital training ranks and he could take no more. He desperately missed his research, his journals and his time with Catherine in the quiet dissectory. Though he despised the plodding, rudimentary nature of his current assignment, his talk with Gussie convinced him that he must find his passion once again. *And that, he would.* He only hoped that Catherine's tea with Lady Cavendish this day would bring her pleasure, as well.

"God's bollocks, Haggett!" cursed Dr. Palgrave, hearing the pitiful cries of the workman from across the great hall. "McKensie, is it too much to ask that your swotter's keep from crippling the patients we are trying to heal?" shouted Palgrave, as he struggled to hold a leather basin steady under the spurting cut in the arm of a rebellious, blood-letting patient.

All heads in the hall turned toward Simon and the howling workman. A public dressing down was exactly the excitement that the bedridden patients cooped up in St. Bartholomew's Hospital lived for. The nervous student finally broke down in tears and ran from the room to the jeers and insults that fanned the flames of the unfortunate situation. Simon cringed at Palgrave's public castigation and, infuriated, prayed yet again for Father Hardwicke's swift return.

The battered administrator had indeed begun to recover and was now permitted to look upon his paperwork for nearly an hour each day. The nuns saw to it, however, that he was kept quiet in his bedstead and visitors were most certainly not allowed. *But, this day, Simon had a plan.* Tucked deep in the pocket of his tunics was a small bottle of Augier brandy from the sleepy little village of Cognac, just to the north of Bordeaux in France. He had slipped the bottle from Cecil's prized wine cellar, with the intention of replacing it as soon as the rebuilding of the Royall Oak Wine Shoppe in the heart of London was completed. He knew that Sister Rosamond attended to Father Hardwicke most days now, and he also knew the good sister dearly liked a wee draught now and again. *Perhaps she could be tempted to bend the rules this once.* Ignoring Palgrave's foul tempered rant, Simon strode from the room, setting one reassuring hand upon the shoulder of the tearful student as he passed. The student lifted his head in anguish.

"I canna' be sent home, Doctor McKensie! I could'na face my father," he cried out. Oswold buried his bright red face in his hands. "He's sacrificed the farm—he's sacrificed everything he has for my medical training. Why, t'would bring him to absolute ruin!"

Simon stopped, his own nerve-rattling first days of training vivid still in his memory. He knelt down to the troubled lad with a rueful smile. "In truth, Oswold, I was desperately shaken myself, the first time I set a bone. Everyone is. Have no fear, ye'll not be sent home."

"But, Doctor Palgrave, sir. He…he terrifies me," admitted the student, embarrassed beyond all measure.

"Ye'll master the technique in no time, I've no doubt. Just stay well clear of Palgrave and ye'll be fine." Simon gave him a nod of encouragement. "Chin up, Haggett, and right back to it—patients await."

Haggett remained where he sat for a moment of baleful contemplations. Small of stature and weak of both chin and muscle, the mere thought of a confrontation with the imposing Palgrave nauseated him no end. He looked up to Simon, then slowly rose and turned for the great hall with a reluctant sigh. "Aye, sir."

Simon grinned and watched him thread his way back to the workman, giving Palgrave a very wide berth. Reaching into his pocket, Simon set a reassuring hand on the bottle once more, then turned, heading toward the stairs that led to the private quarters one floor above.

"Oi!" called the registrar as Simon passed the registration desk.

Still provoked by Palgrave's harsh treatment of the student, Simon was in no mood for this tiresome, little man. He ignored the toady.

"OI!" the registrar bellowed once more.

Simon turned toward the irritating screech. "Did you wish to speak to me?" he asked, with excessive politeness.

The registrar did not answer. Instead, he took a thick packet and flung it toward Simon. "Fer you."

Simon caught the packet and looked down at the measured calligraphy on the escutcheon. *Oxford University.* His heart started to pound. Simon turned from the registrar's desk and found a quiet corner in the now abandoned dissectory. He sank to a bench and stared for a moment at the bound parcel, addressed to *Simon McKensie, Physick, St. Bartholomew's Hospital.* He was struck by the enormity of the moment. With shaking hands, he untied the knotted strings caught up in blood-red sealing wax. Simon reached inside and pulled a letter, astonishing in both its generosity, as well as its brevity, from the top of a stack of journals and scientific notes. He rifled through the carefully transcribed notes, briefly struck by Wren's detailed illustrations, and then set the journals aside. He carefully unfolded the thick parchment letter.

> *Regarding your inquiry, please find enclosed:*
> *Summative scientific research notes and published journals concerning canis blood exsanguination and subsequent transfusion.*
> *Best,*
> *Lower*

Oxford University
15 September 1666

Simon carefully placed the papers back into the packet and then retied the strings. He rose, feeling the bottle of cognac clunk against his leg, then tucked the packet under his arm and headed for the stairs, more determined than ever.

⸺⸻⸺

Sister Rosamond jerked awake at the sound of heavy boots upon the narrow wooden steps that led up to the private chambers. The well-worn bible she held slid with a clunk onto the scuffed floorboards, splaying the pages wide. Quickly wiping the bit of spittal that had trickled from the corner of her mouth with the back of her wrist, she straightened her raiment and adjusted her leather-framed spectacles, then arose stiffly from the wooden chair where she sat guard to the private chamber. She watched nervously for the body that accompanied the thudding steps. Simon stepped into the hallway, smiling. Sister Rosamond visibly exhaled and bent down to retrieve her good book.

"Oh, Dr. McKensie, ye gave me a quite the fright, ye did," she exclaimed with a small chuckle. She removed her glasses and rubbed her tired eyes. "What can I do fer ye?"

"I'd like to speak with Father Hardwicke." He bent down to her, whispering conspiratorially. "Might you see your way clear to bend the rules and allow me a brief visit?"

A brief, playful scowl passed over her plain features. She shook her finger in mock reprimand. "He's to have no visitors disturbin' his rest."

"But, Sister, is it not true that he this day recuperates well?" teased Simon.

"Aye'n 'tis the quiet that's brought him right 'round, indeed." Sister Rosamond smiled and waved toward the stairs. "Away with ye, nae," she yawned. Simon looked closely at the dark circles rimming her eyes.

"I suppose ye've had precious little sleep since the attack," continued Simon, ignoring her orders.

"Ah, a good night's slumber…" she said, with a wistful sigh. She straightened her skirts, then caught his gaze and smiled. "T'would gladden the heart, indeed."

"Then, perhaps I might offer wee curative remedy," winked Simon. He reached into his pocket and withdrew the little bottle of cognac. "Elixir of the gods, you might say." He held it toward her. "For restorative purposes, of course."

Sister Rosamond nearly swooned at the sight. For a brief

moment, her eyes sparkled as she contemplated the exquisite taste of the sweet, fortified wine upon her tongue. She glanced both ways down the hallway, and then held out her hand, palm up. "I s'ppose I could conduct a bed check downstairs," she allowed. Simon pressed the bottle firmly in her hand. Sister Rosamond quickly tucked it into the pocket of her black robes and headed for the stairs. "Five minutes, an' not one second more," she warned. At the top step, she turned back. "Not a' one."

Simon walked twenty paces down the dark hallway to a low-planked door and knocked softly. It had been weeks since Simon had seen the man who, though strict, had recognized the spark of raw intelligence in him from the start. The man who had encouraged his wide-ranging experiments and fed his insatiable intellect and scientific curiosity. *The man who had banished him to a small village where he had found, against all reason, the very life he had been looking for.*

"Enter," bade the faint, reedy voice Simon knew so well.

Simon pushed down on the latch and, ducking his head, stepped into the small, dimly lit chamber. He was startled to see Father Hardwicke laying small on a feather mattress, now a much thinner, deeply aged man. Heavy linens covered a small paned window, darkening the sparsely furnished room. A single candle burned in turned wooden holder on a table next to the rope bedstead. Simon quickly regained his composure. Father Hardwicke turned his head and smiled.

"Good to see you, lad," he whispered, hoarse from the lack of use. He took the packet Simon held toward him. He furrowed his brow, curious. "What have you, then?"

"It's come, Father." Simon could hardly contain himself. "A reply from Oxford. 'Tis from Sir Richard Lower, himself!" His allotted time short, Simon spoke rapidly as he proffered the pages. "I have not fully examined the research, but Father, I wish…I wish to conduct an experiment in blood transfusion."

Father Hardwicke raised himself upon his pillows and stared

at the young man, as he contemplated the lad's extraordinary proposal. He had seen this fire and fierce intelligence in Simon many times before and he was once again in awe. *Truth be told, it made the old priest feel more alive just to be in the presence of the lad.* Father Hardwicke leafed through the papers, thoughtfully musing over the prospect. "Go on."

"You see, Father, I believe that such a procedure could help patients whose blood has been lost in such direful quantities as to cause mortal injury. Consider the possibilities if we were able to put blood back into the body in such equal amounts as had been lost? Might that not reverse the inevitability of death?"

Father Hardwicke contemplated the idea, as he perused Wren's diagrams, fascinated by the science of it. He glanced to Simon. "You, of course, have my permission to conduct any experiment you see fit in your dissectory." Father Hardwicke returned his attention to the research, his old mind captured by the simple elegance of the speculation. "Have you taken measures toward such an experiment?"

Simon caught his breath. "Perhaps you are unaware?"

"Unaware? Of what?"

Simon drew a deep breath and considered his next words, weighing the dreadful consequences he would face, should Dr. Palgrave think he bore witness against him. But God's thunder, Simon could abide the old fool no longer. *The miserable, old thickwit Palgrave is near as sharp as a sack of bricks.*

Father Hardwicke looked up, expectantly. "Out with it."

Exhaling, Simon resigned himself to his fate. He spoke candidly. "Dr. Palgrave, as acting Head Administrator, dismantled the dissectory nearly two months ago. He has demoted me to a position supervising none but the incoming medical students."

Father Hardwicke's eyes widened, then blazed with fury as he worked to absorb the treachery. He gripped the sheets in frustration. "By what right does he conduct such a course?!"

Simon hesitated a moment. "He considers my research… my experiments, to be a blasphemous, mortal sin against God." The priest exploded. "I am still in charge of this hospital!" He caught his breath in a vain attempt to calm himself. "This is untenable beyond all measure," he fretted. "He does not confer with me. I am isolated up here. Why, I am allowed to rise from this bed but twice a day—and only with permission from a…a woman!" he sputtered. Father Hardwicke pounded the bed. "I should have discharged him years ago, but the administrative board, against all protest, shares his religious philosophies." He shook his head in frustration. "I will tolerate it no more! "

Simon refrained from speaking further. He was certain to face unpleasant retribution from Dr. Palgrave for even this day entering Father Hardwicke's room. He did not wish to add to his mounting troubles.

A knock at the door interrupted their conversation. Sister Rosamond looked in. "'Tis time."

Father Hardwicke collected himself and exhaled. He smoothed the sheets to settle his foul mood, and then handed the packet back to Simon.

"I'll see to this."

Simon nodded. He took the papers in hand, and quickly ducked from the room. Sister Rosamond followed him out, closing the door softly behind her. Father Hardwicke lay in the darkened room for a moment as his blood began to boil. Then, with a surge of energy coursing through his veins, he sat up. Throwing the coverings back from the bed, Father Hardwicke set his feet to the floor. *Enough.*

CHAPTER TWENTY-TWO

"CUSTOM, WHEN IT IS INVETERATE, HATH A MIGHTY
INFLUENCE: IT HATH THE FORCE OF NATURE ITSELF."
~ BATHSUA MAKIN

Cavendish Hall
St. James Parish, London
29 October 1666

ady Catherine McKensie," intoned the smartly dressed
butler of Cavendish Hall over the excitable murmurings
of a small group of women. Catherine stood with the butler at
the entrance to the withdrawing room and caught her breath
at the sight of one of the most intriguing chambers she had
ever seen in a city mansion. The arched, barrel ceiling that ran
the length of the gallery was finished in hundreds of wooden,
carved acanthus leaf squares stained a warm chestnut brown.
'Tis as glorious as a piece of hand-cut jewelry. The floor was laid
with golden Cotswald limestone, and two immense stone
hearths set directly opposite one another along the sides of the
gallery, each inglenook blazing with a well-laid fire against the
cool autumn air, were so generously sized that a man could
walk straight into the fireboxes without having to bend down.
The parallel fires created a welcoming warmth to the long
gallery and cast a flickering glow upon the gold-lettered spines
of the books contained in the impressive bespoke library cases
that lined the walls.

At the far end of the chamber, below an immense Gothic
arched, leaded glass window, four plumed hats gathered close
over a set of parchments that lay upon a large desk lifted as one
at the sound of the butler's voice. For a brief moment, Catherine

felt a strange sense of unease, for although she clutched the hand-lettered invitation tightly in her gloved hand, she was terribly intimidated. The butler glanced at Catherine and nodded, then quietly backed away from the doorway.

From behind the desk, a soft voice called out. "Lady McKensie. Welcome to our Thursday gathering." Margaret Cavendish, Duchess of Newcastle-Upon-Tyne emerged from the group in a vibrant swath of rustling fabric. Catherine stared in awe having never before seen such a costume, this one a witty gown of gathered ruby red and raspberry striped silks topped by a shawl of embroidered golden flowers. She was mesmerized by the fantastical design of the frock, much as she had been by the gown Lady Cavendish wore the day they met in the publishing house. It was as though her hostess employed exuberant fashion, rather than exuberant speech, to express her most deeply held artistic impulses.

Lady Cavendish hurried to greet her guest. Speaking softly, but decisively, she took Catherine by the crook of the elbow and led her back toward the women. "Please join us." As they walked the length of the gallery, Catherine took in the elegant, yet bold costumes of the women as they approached the desk. "May I present Lady Phillipa Dillworth, Lady Elizabeth Wilbraham, Miss Bathsua Makin and Miss Aphra Behn," gestured Lady Margaret.

To Catherine's great relief, the ladies all smiled, each nodding a warm welcome. "We stand on no ceremony here, Catherine—may I call you Catherine?" asked Margaret in her whispery voice.

Catherine nodded. "Please."

"We find our formal titles to be cumbersome and unnecessary when we are together, and in that light," she said, gesturing once again, "may I introduce you to Pippa, Bathsua, Aphra, Elizabeth, and," pointing to herself, "of course, Margaret. You don't mind, do you?"

"No…I don't mind," said Catherine, surprised, but strangely comforted by the instant familiarity. "I am very pleased to meet you all."

Margaret reached for a small bell sitting upon the desk. A high-pitched, delicate chime summoned the butler, who appeared in the doorway. "We shall take our tea now." The butler nodded once again and disappeared. Within minutes, a maid entered the room carrying a large silver tray with tea and sweet biscuits. "Set it here," said Margaret, clearing a place at the desk. "I will pour."

"Yes, Milady," said the maid. She set the tray down and left the room.

Margaret poured, and then handed the ceramic vessels in turn to the women, who continued to study the drawings that covered nearly every inch of the broad, walnut-veneered desk. Catherine had never taken tea under such casual circumstances. *She found she rather liked it.* Catherine tilted her head sideways, trying to make sense of the upside down image drawn on the fine-grain parchment paper.

"Have you seen architectural renderings before, Catherine?" asked Elizabeth.

Catherine paused, thinking. "No, I was quite young when our London home was built. I do not recall seeing the plans."

The sure, straight lines, the precise angles and the swooping curves laid out on the paper were tantalizing to her artistic eye. Arched windows placed in perfect symmetry on a columned façade, as many on one side of the entrance as on the other, sparked in her imaginings. The windows on the floors above were smaller but no less symmetrical. She watched as Elizabeth took a straightedge in hand and made a minor shift on one of the landscape parterres, and then made the exact same shift on the opposite side. The top left-hand section had been meticulously filled in with stone and brick elements. The remainder of the drawing had yet to be completed in finishing detail.

"This is a proposal for the addition of wings to Berkshire House, meant for the Duchess of Cleveland, the King's…ah, the King's favored… companion," said Elizabeth, delicately. "It is designed in the Palladian style."

"And the King himself is to approve the plans," said Aphra. "But, of course he will…"

"…Of course he will approve of anything to keep her happy," interrupted Pippa, leaning over the papers. She lifted her head and gave a sidelong glance toward Aphra. "Except perhaps refrain from the theater…"

"Does he enjoy the theater?" asked Catherine, in all innocence.

Pippa set a hand aside her mouth, whispering loudly. "If a certain comedienne by the name of Nell Gwyn is in performance, he does."

"Hush, Pippa," scolded Elizabeth. "The less one knows, the better. 'Tis but a fiction at present," she murmured.

"And yet, if she accommodates the fiction, she shall be rewarded handsomely with much larger quarters," said Aphra, patting the plans with just a touch of dry wit.

"It is said that the king intends to send his yacht to both Flanders and Paris to furnish the palace's grand chambers with furniture, tapestries, mirrors and tableware," offered Bathsua. "That should quickly smooth any aggrieved affections."

"Is there a chamber grand enough for her gaming tables?" Pippa groused.

Bathsua turned to Catherine and whispered. "Pippa was bested by the Duchess the last time they played piquet. Once again, poor Pippa lost a great sum of money."

"With the King overlooking my hand, there was no question as to the outcome of my wager," Pippa pouted. "My husband was quite vexed at him."

Catherine felt very out of place. These women were surprising at every turn.

"Enough now," chided Aphra, ignoring the banter. She

turned her attention back to the proposal. "I am truly in awe, Elizabeth," she said, looking closely at the plans. "It is a graceful and elegant design that will endure the ages. Palladio, himself, would be greatly satisfied by your work."

Catherine furrowed her brow, searching her memory for the reference. "Palladio?"

"The Italian, Andrea Palladio," explained Elizabeth. "He created an architectural style that is rooted in the belief that a universally applied vocabulary of architectural forms is both desirable and possible." She looked carefully at Catherine. "Do you understand?"

Catherine thought fast. "Yes, I...I think I do—would it be a sort of organization of artistic thought? Perhaps it is the defining of a particular aesthetic style from which architects are able to draw upon."

"Exactly," she smiled, as Catherine began to feel more comfortable. "Palladio believed that such a design vocabulary was developed by the ancient Romans, and that careful study and judicious use of those forms will result in beauty." She turned the rendering toward Catherine. "Is his style not beautiful in its mathematical precision and symmetry?"

Catherine studied the drawing with fresh perspective. "It is, indeed, Lady Wil... Elizabeth," she ventured, cautiously.

Elizabeth nodded her approval. "Yes. Please call me Elizabeth."

"Though 'tis a great pity that her name will n'ere be associated with the beauty she creates," said Pippa, crossing her arms in defiant objection.

A look of confusion clouded Catherine's face. "I am afraid I do not understand."

"We women are not meant to use our intelligence nor engage in the professions. Did you not know?" she drawled, arching an eyebrow. "The practice damages the delicate ego of men."

"A caustic wit does not become you, Pippa..." chided Bathsua. Catherine glanced from one woman to another, unsure of the tone being set. "…it becomes me, however," she teased. The women laughed, well accustomed to the clever banterings between friends. Catherine began to laugh herself, suddenly feeling quite at home.

"In all sincerity, however, can you imagine, Catherine?" asked an exasperated Pippa as the laughter died down. "The whole of London has been reduced to rubble and ash by the fire and must needs rebuilding in its entirety. That rebuilding shall require the talents and skills of contractors, stonemasons, woodsmiths, blacksmiths, plasterers and a whole host of laborers—but before *any* such construction can happen, they need the plans. Architectural plans. *From architects.*" She paused, drawing a deep breath, and then continued, holding up a finger for emphasis. "Ahhh, but not from all architects," she cautioned, "from only the *male* of the species…" spat Pippa, utterly disgusted and working herself up to a blaze of righteous indignation. "…for it is not the *custom* of men to acknowledge the intelligence and talents of women."

"Now, Pippa…," cautioned Elizabeth, gently. "We do have a guest."

Margaret turned to Catherine who was watching in open-mouthed fascination, and smiled. "While we encourage lively debate, and in fact, have them often, we do not wish to frighten you with our strong opinions on your first visit." She gave Pippa a slight pat on the arm as a caution to soften her argument.

Having worked herself up to a commendable froth, however, Pippa was not to be silenced. She ignored Margaret's touch. "Do not 'now Pippa' me, Elizabeth Wilbraham," she fired back. "We *all* wish to live our lives with the respect and the freedom to do as we please, just the same as any man."

Bathsua snorted. "We should live er'e long…"

Pippa turned to the group nearly shaking with anger. "You know as well as I that Elizabeth's architectural designs are equal, if not superior, to the men. She has trained under

Pieter Post in Amsterdam, studied the works of Palladio in Italy and *Stradtresidenz* in Germany. She has spent years mastering the art, the science, the mathematics and the engineering of architecture. She is highly qualified, far more then most, and yet she must not sign her name to the work. She must use executant architects to claim credit in *their* name and to supervise construction in her place."

"It really is not equitable," agreed Aphra, joining the vociferous debate.

"And yet, as Pippa says, it is the custom," said Elizabeth.

Bathsua sniffed her displeasure. "Custom, indeed. Simply because something has always been done, does not mean it must needs continue in the same fashion if a better path exists," she spat.

"And exactly what is it you wish me to do?" asked Elizabeth, voicing a modicum of reason. "*Insist* that I claim title to my plans and have not one single workman accept employment to execute the construction—is that what you would want for me? That my plans be consigned to the bottom of a dustbin?"

A rare silence at the simple logic of her argument fell over the group. Margaret moved first.

"Where are my manners?" asked Margaret, smoothing over the awkward moment. She crossed to the bookshelves. "Have I shown you Catherine's book? She has published the most marvelous scientific illustrations of butterflies."

"You own a copy?" asked an astonished Catherine. "I am truly honored," she said, humbled at the kindness shown by such an estimable woman.

"We thought you to be accomplished in some fashion," said Aphra, craning her head to look at the volume. "Margaret often gathers together like-minded women."

The women gathered close around Margaret as she opened the cover to reveal the magnificent illustrations contained inside the pages. Page after page they turned, examining the intricate patterns and markings, the delicate shadings and the sheer variety of butterflies found in England. They looked up at her, then back to the illustrations several times, awed as they were by her artistic talent. Catherine was deeply embarrassed and retreated as far as she could from the women, choosing instead to examine the voluminous collection of books on the shelves. She was relieved beyond measure when the butler came to the door and announced that mid-afternoon dinner was served.

◦∞◦

MaryPryde stifled a sudden sneeze as she opened a glass fronted library cabinet door and flicked a rag across the books. Glimmering dust particles swirled in the late afternoon sunlight that streamed through the library windowpanes. She wiped the minute particles from her eyes and paused a moment to gaze around the wondrous chamber, considering how very fortunate she had been to secure a position in such a fine, stately home. Catherine had been thrilled to see her again, and instantly approved when Gussie hired the girl. In a quiet moment on MaryPryde's first day, Catherine and Simon had taken her aside, privately inquiring about her husband. Though she kept her tongue, Catherine seemed well satisfied to learn that Flynt Pollard had perished in the fire. Oddly, Simon looked as though the weight of the world had been lifted from his shoulders, as well. Though MaryPryde did not understand his reaction, she had been greatly relieved that no more questions had been asked.

Leaning against the cabinet a moment, MaryPryde reveled in the elegant surroundings. She clutched the rag to her chest and fell into her fertile imaginings once more. *The hem of her pale, shell pink gown rustled softly as she walked toward a young man dressed in full, formal regalia. She carried a small bouquet of pastel-tinted sweet peas tied with a silken ribbon that draped nearly to the floor. An admiring crowd gathered close as she stepped into place beside him. She dared a glance. T'was Charles Abbott standing next to her, smiling. He took her hand gently into his own, then, together, they turned to face the minister.* A delicate chime from a French porcelain clock on the library shelf drew her from her fantasies. Just like that, the spell was broken. She chided herself. *He did not even know she was alive.*

In the quiet chamber, she sighed and latched the cabinet door, then opened the next cabinet and flicked the rag once again. The only book in the library that had been turned so that it faced outward, caught her eye, as did the elaborate printing on the hand-bound cover of the book. She read the title. *Butterfly Observations in the Towne of Stockbridge and the Towne of Wells.* She looked closer, not quite believing what else was printed on the cover. *Writ by Lady Catherine Mary Abbott, 1664.* Lady Catherine Abbott? *Could it er'e be possible that Lady McKensie has written an entire book?*

She glanced toward the deserted hallway outside the library. Cedric, Archie and Gussie were occupied elsewhere in the house. She pulled the book from the shelf. Absently setting the rag on the shelf, she opened the cover and read the first page. She looked again toward the empty hallway, and then slid into a seat in one of the leather chairs set before the fireplace. She turned to the next page. So absorbed in the illustrations, she did not hear the footsteps approaching from behind until it was too late.

"Good afternoon, MaryPryde."

The book flew from her hands. MaryPryde instinctively recoiled, the brutal memory of Pollard never far from her thoughts. Charles stood next to her, grinning. "Oh! Beggin' yer pardon, Milord!" she gasped. "I'm ever so sorry…" She jumped to retrieve the book from the floor, and then grabbed her rag, setting the book back on the shelf. Her hands were shaking. *Did he suspect her romantic imaginings?* She glanced toward the hallway, wishing to flee the room.

"For what?" asked Charles, walking to the library case.

"For touching yer possessions. For sitting down." She cast her eyes to the floor. "For looking at the book," she said, softly, embarrassed to have been caught out when she should have been working. *For daring to love you.*

Charles pulled the book back off the shelf and handed it back to her. "Please."

"Oh, no, sir. I couldn't," she said, the flush rising once again in her cheeks.

"Can you not read?" he asked, impulsively.

MaryPryde furrowed her brow. "Aye. I can." She felt vaguely insulted by the redheaded young man standing before her. "My father taught me th' letters," she said, defensively.

"I apologize, I did not mean to offend," Charles faltered, "I only meant…"

"I know what you meant, sir. I am but a serving girl."

"MaryPryde," called Archie, looking in from the hall. "Gussie says 'tis time fer th' bread-makin. Yer needed in the kitchen."

"Aye, Mr. Crawdor," she answered. She turned to Charles and handed the book back. "Thank you, all the same, sir."

His cheeks instantly reddened. *He had put his foot in it.* Charles tried to find the words to make it right, but could only nod. "If you should change your mind…"

MaryPryde snatched the rag back in hand and hurried from the room, biting her lip in embarrassment.

Charles tapped the book in his palm as he watched her leave. *Peculiar girl.*

❦

The ladies sat in the lush garden room of Cavendish House chatting over rose water wafers and tea as several maids cleared the luncheon table. Catherine marveled at the herbs growing in clay pots beneath the arched windows. She immediately recognized the marigold, the sweet bay and the chives, as well as the chamomile that would be used in the household for both medical and culinary purposes. She pointed to a pale, flat-leafed plant with tiny purple flowers and leaned over to Margaret. "May I ask what that plant is?"

"'Tis borage. Useful for the treatment in the yellowing of eyes. We've not had the need, but I confess that I find the study of plants for medicinal purposes fascinating."

Catherine stood and walked to the window for a closer examination of the soft, velvety leaves. She closed her eyes, imagining the strokes upon the paper needed to capture the fine veining and the delicate flowers. She missed putting pen to parchment. *Perhaps she could illustrate a collection of herbs used for healing.*

Bathsua, sneaking one last bite as the maid removed her plate, turned in her chair and faced Catherine. "Do you intend to write another book, Catherine?"

Catherine was startled. It was almost as though Bathsua had divined the very idea turning in her mind. "I have been illustrating a project with my husband in his research at the hospital, but that research has come to an abrupt end, so for the moment, I am idle."

Elizabeth suddenly rose from the table and walked into the library. She returned with Catherine's book. She leafed through the pages. "You have a singular artistic talent.' She glanced up to Catherine. "Have you an eye for figures? Algebra? Geometry?"

"I was tutored in both algebra and geometry and earned the highest marks in both. I was taught science and philosophy, as well."

"Come with me," she said, with a smile. Catherine and the other women followed her back into the withdrawing room and over to the desk. Elizabeth turned the parchment renderings around and pointed to the completed section of the drawing. "Can you see what I have begun up here in the top corner? The finishing details?"

"Yes."

"Do you think you could replicate those details?"

"Yes, I believe I could."

Pippa instantly seized upon the possibilities. "With all of the rebuilding in London, Elizabeth has more work than she can entertain…"

"…and yet, I can't bear to turn the opportunities away," finished Elizabeth. She hesitated a moment. "Would you consider taking on the project? It is quite tedious and time-consuming, and there is a deadline of mid-March, but perhaps you might enjoy the work?"

In that very moment, her restlessness dissipated. "Yes, Elizabeth. I would very much like that, indeed."

CHAPTER TWENTY-THREE

17 Cock Lane
Farringdon Without
Smithfield, London
1 December 1666

Dr. Palgrave, balancing a cloth-covered plate of food in one hand and a mangy cat in the other, kicked open the door to his boardinghouse room with his scuffed boot. Ducking beneath the low opening, he entered the darkened room and set the plate atop a splintered, unsteady wooden table. The cat jumped from his arms and padded across the floorboards, on the prowl for a mouse that had rustled behind a cabinet. Palgrave struck a flint to a candle stub on the table, illuminating the bleak, filthy room, then crossed to the chamber pot at the foot of his bedstead, kicking several cats away from the rim. He did his business, then grabbed the pot and opened the small, paned casement window above it. "Oi!" he bellowed, leaning out over the transom. "Gardy-loo!" Without waiting, he threw the contents out onto the narrow, fog-shrouded lane below. He let the cold air clear the foul, animal stench from the room for a moment, then rewound the latch and shut the window. Palgrave set the pot back in the corner, and then, shoving several more cats off the table, sat down to the lukewarm stew prepared by his landlady. Spitting on a knife to clean the dried bits off, he took a bite and grunted at the cold, gray meat. He set the knife down and shoved the plate aside. He had no appetite. Nine scrawny cats leapt smoothly to the tabletop and, crowding around the plate, devoured every last morsel.

Sent down. And, not just sent down, but flung so far down since Hardwicke's return that he was now allowed authority over none but the first year bonesetters. For Father Hardwicke had indeed returned with a vengeance, enraged that Palgrave had seized upon his administration offices without permission, enraged that he had taken a personal revenge upon Simon and dared demote the hospital's best physician, and especially enraged that he had not once taken counsel with Hardwicke during the long recovery. Most egregious of all, Hardwicke was furious that Palgrave had dismantled Simon's dissectory. Palgrave had seethed privately over the exile for weeks, but this night something was different. *Very different.* For he had at last laid witness to the remaining research stored in the anteroom off Hardwicke's chamber. *And he had seen it all.*

With plenty of time to think in the long, painfully dull weeks since being demoted, Godfrey Palgrave had devised a plan. He had this day waited until Father Hardwicke was well engaged with patients, and then Palgrave had slipped into the storeroom, at last prying open every single wooden crate with a feverish desperation that ripped at his senses. He rifled through the contents, staring in utter disbelief. The crude drawings of dead bodies, their insides gutted and splayed godlessly for the world to see. The abhorrent, blasphemous dissections that sickened him to the core. The mendicants—the penniless, homeless beggars violated beyond all righteous decency. He had gripped the fibrous parchments with his swollen, bony knuckles and stared closer, his eyes widening at the sight. *He now knew exactly from whence they came.* A sudden clutch of resentment began to seethe inside Palgrave; a resentment that rapidly built to white-hot fury, for printed in careful script beneath the mendicant notation was a smudged signature. *S. McK. Physick. 25 December 1664* He stared at the date in horror. That this sinful abomination had been performed on the holiest of days inflamed his white-hot hatred all the more.

Palgrave, as Alfred Clarke had before him, fought tooth and nail with the boy since his arrival for medical training four years earlier, and at every last turn, the damnable whelp had bested the both of them. *Why could Hardwicke not see that the discoveries made in treating the plague by this young jackstraw were nothing more than a felicitous stroke of fortune?* In his fury, Palgrave had crushed the parchment with his hands, feeling the paper rip between his shaking fingers. He didn't care. *Lord, how he despised this weanling.* Palgrave had given his life to St. Bartholomew's only to be cast aside the moment a greenhorn showed a fleck of promise. *In all creation above, could Hardwicke not see that the boy's unholy experiments made mockery of not only Father Hardwicke's faith, but of Palgrave's fervent beliefs, as well? Why, the truth of it is that the milksop's sacrilegious enquiries make mockery of God, himself!*

A verminous tabby crawled up into his lap, mewing a soft, plaintive cry. Absently scruffling the cat's ears for a moment, Palgrave suddenly felt very old. He lifted the cat to his face and buried his nose in its soft, patchy fur. The cat flicked him with an affectionate brush of its tail. *He had given the hospital all he had. He had nothing left. He was spent.* Godfrey roughly brushed away an unaccustomed wetness that leaked from the corner of his eyes with his thumb, and then picked up the knife. For a long moment, he examined both sides of the dull, pitted blade. Like that, the smoldering fury he had been nursing for so long suddenly seized hold of his entrails like a swift crack of thunder. The old man gripped the blade, tossed the cat to the floor and with one vicious flick, whipped the knife straight into the wall. It hung there, wavering, much like the biblical rage he felt so very deep in his soul. *Bastard.*

CHAPTER TWENTY-FOUR

"THE PROPER METHOD FOR INQUIRING AFTER THE PROPERTIES
OF THINGS IS TO DEDUCE THEM FROM EXPERIMENT."
~ SIR ISAAC NEWTON

Bealeton House
St. James Parish, London
4 December 1666

Simon warmed himself before a fire blazing in the library's stone hearth, examining the notes and journal entries sent from Sir Richard Lower once again. He had prepared for weeks, methodically assembling the tools he would need, planning the methods he would employ. He had this day paid for a sheep's bladder and a flacon of sheep's blood to be delivered from the butcher at the hour of the experiment, and on the walk home, Simon purchased several of the fattest quills sold at Minerva-Poole Stationers, Ltd., just off Fetter Lane. Though most of the West End shops had been shuttered for weeks from the smoke and structural damage caused by the fire-break explosions, the resolute stationer had managed to reopen his establishment just days after the inferno. Stoking the coals with an iron poker, Simon thought of the proper, meticulously dressed stationer fussing over the merchandise as though he had any competition left. He nearly laughed aloud at their exchange earlier in the day.

The shop bell clanging had announced Simon's arrival. "How may I assist you, sir?" William Poole asked, straightening the sheaves of heavy parchment papers that hung over a wooden rack next to the tidy shop desk.

Simon blew into his fists, warming his cold fingers, and then sifted carefully through a clay container of goose quills that sat on a table by the door. "I should like to buy a quill with a large hollow for a scientific experiment."

His interest piqued, the stationer drew closer. "What sort of experiment, sir? I only ask, of course, so that I might better assist you."

"A blood transfusion. From a sheep."

The stationer caught his breath, momentarily taken aback. His eyes widened. "You wish to do what with it, sir?" he coughed. He had cleared his throat, still not quite understanding the proposal.

"I intend to use the quill to transfer the blood of a sheep into the arm of a man," grinned Simon, amused at the momentary expression of shock that crossed the man's face. "I therefore wish to purchase a quill with the widest of barrels. Several of them, in fact."

The stationer had fallen silent in pensive contemplation of the unusual enterprise, and then quickly regained his composure. "I see. One moment, please." The shopkeeper disappeared into the rear of the building. He had re-emerged moments later, carrying a vast tray of feathered goose quills. "Perhaps one of these might suit your needs," he said, setting the tray on the shop table.

And three of them had indeed suited Simon's needs. He had chosen the fattest quills from the lot. On impulse, he bought Catherine a pretty illustration quill pen with a gold filigree hilt as a Christmas gift. He tucked the package into the pocket of his tunics as he left the store. Simon wrapped his cloak tighter and turned down the narrow, cobbled lane for the long, cold walk home.

Simon laid the notes and a stack of leaflets advertising for a volunteer on a wide table, then settled back into a leatherhide chair by the hearth and closed his eyes. He laid his head against the back of the chair, satisfied at last that he had done all he could. He had reviewed the notes on the procedure for weeks. His tools were ready. The restored dissectory was ready and Father Hardwicke had given his approval. All he needed now was the patient. To that end, he had also purchased a small notice in the London Gazette with the offer of three crowns wages for the duration of the experiment. The notice would be published in the following week's edition. He had arranged for a boy to circulate the leaflets on the lanes of Smithfield. *He was ready.*

He felt a kiss brush across his hair. He opened his eyes. The leather creaked beneath him as he turned and looked up. Catherine stood above him laughing. She held a large, bound set of parchment papers in her arms. He could not help but stare, for the cold air outside had heightened the bright pink flush in her cheeks. He was taken aback once again by her delicate beauty. *Ahhh, but 'tis deceptive, that beauty, for it masks the rare intelligence and kindness that enthralls the aching soul far more.*

"My apologies if I startled you," she said, perplexed by his steady gaze.

He smiled, then reached up and pulled her into his lap. The papers fell to the floor. "Ahhh, Cassie m'lassie," he teased, "are ye not completely bewitching? Circe herself could not captivate a man's heart more." He nuzzled her neck and played with the bow at the back of her gown, giving it a slight pull.

Catherine sat straight up. Simon recoiled and instantly dropped the silken fabric. *What had he done? Had he pressed his attentions too far?* "Forgive me," he whispered, confused once again by women's ways. He cast about desperately for something to do to relieve the awkward moment. He reached for the leaflet, pretending to review the notice.

"No, no, Simon!" she reassured him. "An apology is not necessary. I was just startled." For a moment, she seemed lost in a memory. "Cassie m'lassie," she said, softly." My father used to call me by that name."

Simon exhaled with visible relief. "I was born up near the Scottish border where everyone is a lassie or laddie. I suppose it comes naturally," he explained, his blue eyes crinkling at the thought.

"Well, I like it." She took the paper and placed it back on the table, then leaned in and kissed him tenderly on the lips.

"Perhaps we might retreat upstairs," he murmured, his lips exploring hers, his fingertips tracing the slow curve of her gown.

"Perhaps the door could be locked," she whispered back, nibbling his ear.

Simon blinked his eyes wide in surprise, then instantly rose and set her on the hearth. Hastening to the heavy wooden door, he swung it shut and set the iron latch, then bent down to look closer. "There is no lock." Simon straightened and turned back at the sound of her laughter.

"More's the pity," teased Catherine, with a playful glint in her eyes.

"I'll see to you later," he said, teasing her back. The parchments lying on the floor caught his notice. "My apologies, Catherine. My attentions these last weeks have been to the experiment, I fear I've not paid heed to your pursuits. What have you there?"

She reached for the bundle and untied the twine, then spread the parchments across the table with an excitable grin. "Columns."

He looked confused. "I beg your pardon?" He sat back down and looked closer in the firelight.

She shifted the papers. "Lady Wilbraham has been teaching me architectural theory. I had no idea there was so much to it. Such as how to site the home to take advantage of not only the warmth, but the coolness of the sun, or how to direct the heat of the kitchen to the living space, and yet, maintain distance enough to protect from fire. There is so much I hadn't thought of, it's as if an entirely new world existed that I knew nothing about."

"I hadn't thought of such things, myself."

Catherine pointed to a complex illustration. "Today, she taught me to render columns. In Palladio's architectural vocabulary, there are specific geometric calculations to their swellings and dimunations."

Simon's eyes widened. She had spoken but two sentences and he was already baffled. "Their swellings and dimu's...what?"

"Dimunations." She laughed, pulling her brand new copy of Palladio's *"I Quattro Libri dell 'Architettura"* from the bookshelf. Leafing to one of the first sections, Catherine pointed to a detailed drawing. "You see? The higher the column is, the less it must needs diminish toward the top, because the height, by reason of the distance, has that effect."

"I'm afraid I do not understand," said Simon, shaking his head in puzzlement.

She outlined the column with her finger. "This particular drawing illustrates the exact way the columns ought to be formed, If you look closely, the diameter of the uppermost part of the column must needs be smaller than at the bottom, with a kind of a swelling in the middle." Simon was attempting to absorb that complex information when she pointed to a calculation on the opposite page. "You see, this shows mathematically that if the column is fifteen feet in height, the thickness at the bottom will be divided into six and one half parts, five and a half of which will be the thickness for the top."

Simon groaned. "Aye! Stop… I beg of you, please stop!" He grinned and wrapped his arms around her slender waist, pulling her close. "The study of anatomy is far, far easier to understand." Nuzzling her cheek, Simon closed the book and clumsily set it to one side of the chair. In the quiet of the timbered library, a vast pile of logs on the iron grate broke apart. The fire erupted, blazing with a hot intensity. Sparks shot from the crackling flames. Simon held her tightly and kissed the back of her neck. "However, confounded by the calculations as I may be, I am perfectly willing to be set straight no matter how much practice it may take," he murmured.

"Are you speaking of geometry?" she whispered, turning as their lips met in the warmth of the firelight.

"Perhaps…" he said, kissing her again. "Perhaps not."

She sighed contentedly and laid her head upon his shoulder. He absently played with her hair, reveling in the soft touch of her skin upon his own. He wound a tendril around his fingers, admiring the bright sheen of copper backlit by the flames, and then kissed her once more, a kiss so deep and tender that sent shivers coursing down his spine. He clung to her as a man would to a sailing ship's life ring. A quiet knock at the entrance to the library broke the spell.

"Am I interrupting?" teased Charles, peeking into the room.

"Nae," laughed Simon, dropping her curl. He rose from the chair and extended his hand in greeting.

Catherine reluctantly stood and straightened her skirts. "Yes, you are!" she grinned, tying her unruly waves back into the velvet ribbon that bound them up.

"My apologies, indeed," laughed Charles, unapologetic in the least. He dropped his lanky frame into the companion leather chair by the fire and threw his long legs upon the hearth to warm his boots.

Simon stood fully, offering his chair to Catherine.

"Thank you," she smiled. "Charles has clearly forgotten his manners."

"Nae, I have done nothing of the kind," protested Charles. "Forgive me, Catherine, it has been a rather eventful day," he said, chagrined. He rose and pulled a wooden library chair closer and gestured to the comfortable leather chair. "Please, Simon."

Charles tipped the wooden chair onto its back legs, stretching his back. "Gussie says that supper will be served in a half hour's time, and all's the better, for I am absolutely famished."

MaryPryde brought a tea service into the library and, setting it on the side table, began to pour. "Gussie thought you might like a bit of tea to warm yourselves, Milady," she said, as she gave Catherine a cup. The leaflets on the table caught her eye. She leaned in closer to read the notice. She glanced to Simon, then back to the stack of papers. *An idea began to form.* She quietly slipped a leaflet into the pocket of her apron.

"Thank you, MaryPryde," said Catherine, gratefully taking a

sip of the hot brew. MaryPryde poured two more cups, handing first one to Simon, then the other to Charles. She turned back to the table for a moment, set her own hands on the porcelain.

Simon stood once more and warmed his hands before the fire. "What has made your day so eventful, if I may ask?"

"I have had a letter from Uncle George." Charles hesitated a moment. "He has offered to stake my scholarship to a university in the colonies called Harvard. He writes that Boston is growing, and educated men of all professions are desperately needed, most especially solicitors, physicks and land agents. If that does not appeal, he offers a position in his shipping company." He furrowed his brow in thought. "I suppose that Uncle has taken it upon himself to stand in Father's stead with regard to my future."

MaryPryde caught her breath. She set the teapot on the tray with a clunk. Heads turned sharply at the sound. "I beg your pardon," she murmured as she quietly took up the tray.

"Have you given weight to his proposal?" asked Simon.

"Indeed, I have considered it heavily, and today, I have come to a decision." He took a deep breath. "I have decided to forestall a career in navigation," he said, to a near audible sigh of relief from MaryPryde as she took her leave.

"But you have always loved the sea!" exclaimed Catherine. "What has changed your mind?"

Charles stood. Turning his back to the fire, he faced them and spoke in earnest. "T'was the hanging of Hubert in Tyburn last month, Catherine." He began to pace before the hearth, his hands clenched with passion. "I cannot stop thinking of the spectacle. Before that hour, I could not have even once conceived of such a wicked thirst for blood. But by my oath, that day I laid witness to hundreds of vengeful citizens crowding the gallows square, each to a man chanting with glee to witness the most gruesome of sights." He suddenly stopped pacing, his color high with emotion. "Men. Women. Children, even, shouting for the death of what was quite possibly an innocent man," he said, still shaken by the memory. "I confess I was sickened by the very sight of it. It is said that the judge himself bore direct witness to the King as to Hubert's derangement, though none, including the king, stood in defense of the wretched man. In the end, none could save him."

Tears sprang to Catherine's eyes at the thought. "Oh, Charles, the poor man," she whispered.

"Aye. I confess that I did not follow the trial, but how could the judge proceed if even there were the slightest possibility of hanging an innocent soul?" asked Simon in disbelief. "How could no one stand to his defense?"

"T'was like the desperate French woman during the fire, murdered before my eyes by a vengeful crowd merely upon an accusation. One single voice shouting above the mob. One reckless indictment cast with no proof whatsoever! Justice was not served to either soul." Charles' reddening cheeks and clenched fists betrayed his passion and deep sense of honor. He took a steadying breath. "Why, Bloodworth has yet to stand trial for his privations during the early hours of the fire, though enraged Londoners cry for his head, as well. And that is why I have declined Uncle George's offer." He played with the edges of the architectural renderings for a moment as he gathered his courage. "I intend to remain in England. I have applied to Lincoln's Inn, one of the Four Inn's of Court, to undertake the study of law." He turned to Catherine and Simon once more, a determined set to his chin belaying more bravado than perhaps he felt. "I received my acceptance today."

Simon jumped to his feet, offering his hand in congratulations. "Well done, Charles! Well done."

Charles ducked his head in embarrassment. "Thank you, Simon."

Catherine jumped from the chair to hug her brother. "Father would be proud of your decision and I know Aunt Viola will be much relieved to have you here in England, and safely on land." She stepped back to look at her brother standing tall before her in a way he never had before. He was a man grown and it had happened in the blink of an eye. "Perhaps a taste of champagne would be in order?"

Charles' eyes widened in surprise at the offer. "Champagne?"

She smiled and reached for the bell to summon MaryPryde.

A sudden pounding at the doorway to the mansion startled the three from their celebrations. They ran from the library at the urgent blows to the knocker. The butler opened the door to an anxious young man who proffered a folded note.

"Cedric?" called Catherine, hurrying into the entry hall. She could feel an inexplicable dread rising.

"'Tis Jock, from the Abbey," he called. Cedric examined the letter. "For you, Milady," he said, handing her the missive.

"It is from Aunt Viola," she said, tearing into the waxed seal with shaking hands. She read the missive, and then crushed it to her chest. "The mayor."

Simon took the letter and smoothed it out.

> *The mayor has taken seriously ill. You must return to the Abbey in all haste, for I fear the worst.*
> *V.*

CHAPTER TWENTY-FIVE

"IS NOT THIS HOUSE AS NIGH HEAVEN AS MY OWN?"
~ SIR THOMAS MORE

Abbottsford Abbey
Stockbridge, Buckinghamshire
5 December 1666

The gentle, rolling hills of Buckinghamshire stretched before them as the faint light of dawn rose pink above the distant forests. The horses had picked their way slowly over the road from London toward the little village of Stockbridge with nothing but the soft glow of a lantern and the wink of an alabaster moon between scudding clouds to light the way. Soft clops and the rhythmic swaying of the coach through the long night had lulled its three exhausted passengers into a fretful sleep.

The carriage lurched in a deep rut, jostling Catherine awake. She glanced to a still sleeping Charles and Simon, and then rubbed her tired eyes, trying once more to prepare herself for what she might find at the Abbey. *God willing the mayor survives the affliction that has befallen him, for it would be cruel in the extreme for Aunt Viola to have waited a lifetime for love, then have it last but a single twelvemonth.*

Catherine leaned her head against the side of the carriage and sighed at the melancholy thought of her aunt in mourning. Her warm breath left a vaporous cloud upon the cold window. Wiping the fog with her gloves, Catherine looked through the glass. The clouds had at last cleared and before her lay the wondrous sight of a fresh layer of sparkling snow blanketing the fields. *She was home.* The familiar sight of the valley began to soothe her troubled thoughts. Cold, frosty air seeping into the coach made her shiver. Pulling the pile of thick quilts close, Catherine snuggled deeper into Simon's arms. He idly scratched where her hair grazed his chin, and then settled himself against the bench before falling back to sleep.

The sun rising over the snow-dusted hills hit the window and caused a sharp glare through the glass. Catherine squinted as the carriage slowed to approach the y-shaped turning for Wells or Stockbridge. A massive slab of limestone that the locals called the boundary stone hung out over the road, casting a wide shadow over the carriage as it passed beneath. In the brief moment of darkness under the monolithic buttress, memories of the plague-year came flooding back to Catherine as though time itself had been suspended. The stone had been the boundary that separated Wells from the rest of the countryside as one by one, the quarantined villagers sacrificed their lives to keep the plague from spreading beyond its borders. Though in number the deaths were few, each lost soul left an unyielding ache imprinted upon her heart. *Her father. Seton, the tailor. The dressmaker, Lisette Chanon. Dear old Maudie. The Barlowe sisters, and the others, thirteen in number, and each known and so very loved in the two villages that nestled together like spoons in the little valley.*

The carriage took a hard right turn at the stone outcropping and headed for the Abbey, just this side of Stockbridge. She briefly wondered if she would find her home much changed in the many months since she had been in London, but as the coach jounced down the long, tree-studded entrance lane, a peculiar feeling began to rise in her thoughts. With a start, she suddenly realized that she missed the city. Not once in her imaginings did she ever think London would take hold of her affections, but something here troubled her greatly. *There is a sadness that clings to the valley, still.* Every hill, every tree, every last field and glen she had loved since childhood reminded her of her father. At times, she missed him so much she thought her heart would shatter.

Sir Alvyn Abbott was a man of remarkable qualities, qualities she feared she could ne'er measure up to. Honest, loyal and kind beyond measure, he endeavored to provide for the people of the valley. *How he cared.* The coaching inn over in Wells, the stableyards where the plague-stricken villagers were treated in isolation, in fact, nearly every building and commerce project undertaken in the valley had been either initiated or financed by Lord Abbott to benefit the villagers and secure their futures. His kindness and generosity knew no bounds, and yet she knew in her heart that he had passed from this world into the next with the thought that he had not once in his life done enough.

She looked to Simon, still sleeping on the bench beside her. Catherine gazed at his strong, sure profile and marveled that he was cut from exactly the same cloth as her father. *Such a fine man was rare, indeed.* She remembered with disgust the coward she had nearly married. *Miles Houghton.* He had selfishly run from the quarantine, escaping to France, while Simon had stayed, working selflessly through the long days and nights for months to save as many souls as he possibly could. Though she well knew Miles to be irresponsible and shallow, she had not known the extent of his character until the day he ran from the quarantine, nor had she truly known the depths of her own heart until the plague forced her hand. *T'was the death of her father that had given her courage enough to chart her own path rather than the path Aunt Viola had chosen for her in childhood.* Tears flooded her eyes as she thought of the last words her father spoke aloud. *You must do everything you wish in this life.* Even as he lay dying, Lord Abbott knew that Miles was not the man for her. *He knew Simon was.*

Through her unfathomable sorrow, Catherine had somehow gathered the courage to take those words to heart. She had broken the engagement to Miles. She had gone to London, butterfly illustrations in hand. She had found a publisher on her own, and most miraculous of all; she had married the kindest, most intelligent soul she had ever met. They had laughed at her all her life, those mean-spirited girls from the village, and yet she had far surpassed them in her accomplishments. Would they know? In an uncharacteristic moment of infinite satisfaction, Catherine found she no longer cared.

"The Abbey, Milady," called out Jock, as he drew the carriage up the crushed stone approach to the massive, herringbone-brick and timbered country house.

To Catherine's surprise, Viola herself opened the heavy, arched door. She was dressed in dark, somber clothing, and for the briefest of heart-stopping moments Catherine indeed feared the worst.

"Come, come," called Viola, waving an urgent hand.

Jolted awake, Simon grabbed his medical kit and followed Catherine and Charles from the carriage. Viola ushered them straight up the carved wooden staircase into the family sleeping quarters. At the far end of the hallway, they entered a quiet chamber and were shocked to see the normally gregarious mayor lying pale in the light of a single candle flame, and still under several layers of heavy quilts. Catherine began to tremble, for the vivid memory of her father lying deathly ill in the coaching inn stall still burned raw. A familiar, searing ache began to take hold. She turned to Simon and buried her face in his cloak, fighting back tears.

"Gather your courage, Catherine, for surely it will be needed," whispered Viola with surprising strength.

Simon stepped to the velvet-canopied bedstead and set his hand upon the mayor's damp brow. "When did this happen, Viola?" he asked, his eyes urgent in deep concern. Simon set his fingers upon the mayor's neck. He shot Catherine a brief, worried glance.

"T'was but two nights ago, Simon. We were nearly finished with supper when Cecil suddenly rose in his chair. He cried out, and then fell to the floor." She winced at the thought.

"T'was a frightening sight, one I'll not long forget." She paused a moment, reliving the episode in her mind. "I called out to him, but he just lay there, hand to chest." The words caught in her throat at the recollection. "Jock carried him up to our chamber and he has lain thusly since. Although he now responds, I fear that he is very, very ill."

Groaning softly, the mayor stirred and tried to open his eyes. Viola reached for a dainty silver dish and set it beneath the candle, then pulled the stopper from a thick glass bottle. Simon looked closer at the mixture of herbs and shimmering, glowing bits of iridescence in the pale light, then watched, transfixed, as she carefully poured a thick liquid from the bottle into the mix and stirred with gentle precision. She dipped the spoon into the concoction then held it to the Mayor's lips. "Here you are, sweetings. Can you take a bit?"

"Stop!" cried Simon, breaking the spell. He reached for the spoon and examined the liquid. "What on earth is this?"

"'Tis a grinding of pearls and sage, mixed with a syrup of rose, saffron and jacinth," said Viola.

Simon looked perplexed. "A grinding of pearls?"

"I had it sent from the apothecary in Gravesleigh. He said it was his finest restorative formulary. I...I gave them my own string."

A flush of anger rose in his face. "Set it aside, Lady Viola," he said, disgusted by the swindling charlatans who preyed upon the innocent and desperate. "'Neither pearls, nor emeralds, nor priceless rubies will cure him.'"

"I would give my jewel box in the entirety if the stones would save my...husband." A tear trickled down her cheek as she whispered the word, as though she still could not believe she was a married woman.

Simon shook his head. "Feckless concoctions, incantations, and foolish superstitions cure no ills, but for the purse of the herbalist who would profit from your adversity," he spat in contemplation of such greed. "'Tis aught but a confluence of science and logic that will cure the mayor of his affliction."

Resigned, she set the spoon on the table. "I do not know what to do," Viola said in soft despair. She turned to Simon; her eyes circled dark with exhaustion. "Can you say what affliction has befallen him?"

Simon rose from the bedside, then walked to the window and pulled the thick tapestries aside. Morning sun flooded the darkened room. He set his hands to the sill and stared out through the leaded glass panes toward the symmetrical, snow-covered topiaries that graced the estate's formal gardens. Deep in thought, he finally turned to Viola and spoke plainly. "His pulse is weak. The pain in the chest, the ashen pallor… I believe it to be either apoplexy or syncope, Milady."

Viola clutched at Catherine's arm. Though it seemed she wished to cry out and faint herself, Viola somehow retained her composure. "My God," she whispered.

Simon looked once more to Catherine, as though questioning whether he should explain further.

Catherine nodded. "We must know what lies ahead."

Simon elaborated. "His affliction looks to be either an episode of apoplexy, a kind of unconsciousness of the mind, or possibly, syncope, a far lesser affliction," he said, gently.

Viola gasped. "My apologies, Simon, I fear I do not understand a word you say," she said, rattled to her very being.

"In the most general sense, Lady Viola, apoplexy 'tis a type of palsy to the body—a…a sudden loss of consciousness resulting in privation of the senses and motion in the nerves, whereas syncope is rather a sudden fainting spell due to a weakening of the heart. Though I fear we cannot say exactly why the heart is weakened."

At that, Viola gave a soft moan and dabbed her eyes with a ruffled handkerchief. After a moment, she collected herself, then lifted her chin and nodded once more. "Go on."

"We will not know which infirmity he suffers from for

several days, perhaps a week. Should a fever arise, his health will be spared, although any return to London would be delayed, for the mayor will need recuperation in the quietude and fresh air of the countryside for several months or more. And if there is no fever..." Simon paused, and took a deep breath, "...I fear his condition is dire."

Viola sank to the bedstead, her head bowed against the news. The mayor groaned softly. Heartbroken, Viola turned and leaned across the thick coverlet. "What is it, sweetings? What would you like?" she asked, tenderly rubbing the top of his hands.

"Water," he whispered, his voice hoarse and low.

As Viola poured a glass from the bedside pitcher, Simon motioned for Catherine to walk with him to the far end of the chamber. "I'll not lie to you, Catherine, he is terribly ill," he whispered.

"Can anything be done?"

"There is nothing to be done but pray for the fevers."

CHAPTER TWENTY-SIX

Abbottsford Abbey
Stockbridge, Buckinghamshire
10 December 1666

Catherine leaned down to the polished sidesaddle, her leg tensing around the pommel, her heart pounding in unbridled exhilaration. Savoring the thick, leather scent mixed with the earthy sweat of her Irish Connemara jumper, she cried out, urging the horse onward. She could hear the ragged breaths and snorts of her mount. She felt the straining, powerful muscles that churned ever closer to an earthwork enclosure at the edge of the estate. Catherine gripped the reins low and tight to the neck as her prized thoroughbred soared over a low fieldstone wall, ice crystals spraying in their wake. Hollow, thudding hoof beats pounded as they charged across a snowy field made fallow by the winter's cold. Clambering up a small embankment to the road that led into the little village of Wells, her cheeks were flushed red in the biting wind, her eyes stung with the cold, her hands were numb inside her fur-lined riding gloves, but she felt none of it. *She felt alive.*

For this one moment, Catherine felt free from the darkness enshrouding the Abbey. Free from the sadness and fear. *Free from the death that seemed to cling to the edges of her life.* Her father. Her friends. And now, possibly, the mayor. Even the abbey itself seemed strangely lifeless, especially at this time of year, for the month of December had always been filled with a whirlwind of gatherings, friends calling, dancing and parties. For the first time in her life, there would be no Christmas feast at Abbottsford Abbey. *Everything feels sad and melancholy.* After sitting with Viola in the mayor's darkened chamber day and night since their arrival, she needed to reassure herself that in the village, people were still laughing, working and living. When Charles offered once more this morning to spell her, Catherine had at last accepted.

Against a leaden sky, the gothic, stone church spire of Wells came into view as she rounded the last bend in the road. "Yah!" she cried out once more. The horse lowered its head and charged forward toward the Royal George Inn, one of seven stops along the coaching road that led to London.

Catherine held a special spot in her heart for the inn that had been financed by her father. During the construction of the Royal George, Sir Abbott had convinced the *Royal Coach Company, Ltd.,* to route the coach road through Wells, thereby ensuring a steady stream of trade, customers and income to the people of the valley. Such concern came as naturally as breathing to him. Catherine felt a small pang of guilt taking the Abbey carriage from London the night they travelled from London, for her father had always insisted they use the public coach, and he would take no quarter. *If the Abbotts' do not use the public coach, why would we expect any of the others?* He had been right, for the coach was always full and trade in town was bustling.

Catherine wheeled her horse into the courtyard of the inn amid flying stones and wet snow and pulled him up short. She looked for the stable hand, and grinned when she saw eleven-year old Toby emerge from the barn. Exhilarated and breathing hard from the ride, Catherine slid to the ground and stood facing the curly-headed lad with her arms open wide.

"Lady Abbott!" he cried, running headlong into her embrace, nearly knocking her over in his excitement.

"'Tis Lady McKensie, nae!" she laughed, hugging him tightly.

"Aw, yes, Miss—I'd heard ye an' Simon were married! "

She rustled his curls, and then held him at arm's length, taking the measure of the boy. "Aye, 'tis grown ye are, Toby. Nearly as tall as I am, indeed!" Toby lifted his chin in an attempt to overtop her. "Not yet, you muggins, not quite yet," she teased. Catherine grew serious for the moment, remembering how Simon had bound his broken leg from the carriage accident the day she and Simon first met, and then saved the boy's life during the plague. "How are you, Toby?"

"I am well, your Ladyship," he grinned, taking the reins in hand. He led the horse toward a small stable in the courtyard. "Barely a limp."

"Glad to hear it, Toby," she said, genuinely relieved that there had been no lingering effects. "And your studies? Are you still working with Master Howell?"

"Aye, Milady, everyday after chores. Miss Flossie sees to it. She has a daughter, Molly, an' we both ride to the Abbey for lessons. She wants Molly to be a fine lady, 'an I still intend to be a physick, just like Simon. A' course there are no lessons while the Lord Mayor is unwell."

"Miss Flossie?" asked Catherine.

"The lady that took Miss Maudie's place after she died o' the plague. You remember Miss Maudie?"

"I do remember Maudie, Toby," said Catherine, "but I have not yet met Miss Flossie."

"You'll like her, Milady." He leaned toward her and whispered. "She walks about with the butcher, Master Eldrick," he grinned. "Master Eldrick sometimes gives me extra lamb to put in the dinner pot, now."

"Well, now, I shall have to meet your Miss Flossie!" laughed Catherine as she straightened her cloak. "Perhaps a cup of tea might warm my hands," she winked. Catherine handed Toby a small silver coin, then walked across the brick courtyard toward the inn. Though she tried to avert her eyes, she could not help but glance down the hill to the expansive stableyard where Simon had quarantined those ill with the plague. *Where her father had died.* Simon's extraordinary measures had saved so many in the village when he endeavored to isolate the sick from the well. For months, he alone had kept the plague from spreading further in the village and beyond its borders. She furrowed her brow and stared at the compound. *Something looks different.* She suddenly realized that the row of stables they had used for the plague victims had been burned to the ground. The other stablerows looked different to her, as well. *They looked deserted.*

Catherine entered the familiar, low-ceilinged entrance hall of the coaching inn, rubbing her gloves together to warm her hands.

"Good afternoon, Milady!" called out a woman from the crowded public room. She scuttled into the hall and helped Catherine remove her cloak.

"Good afternoon," answered Catherine, shrugging the heavy woolen cape from her shoulders. "Might I trouble you for some tea?"

"Ahh, an' 'tis no trouble, t'all. Follow me, if ye would, please," said the woman, hanging the cloak on a peg by the door. She led Catherine past the raucous public room and into a quieter, more refined private room that was reserved for the wealthier patrons.

Catherine chose a table by the hearth and removed her riding gloves to warm her hands above the fire burning behind an iron screen. Milk-painted paneling in a soft mustard color and the lit iron-forged candle chandelier hanging from the ceiling created a welcoming atmosphere. Catherine instantly felt the tension in her shoulders ease.

"Flossie's th' name," the woman said, with a broad, welcoming smile.

Catherine was drawn to the warmth that seemed to exude from the woman with golden skin and hair the color of nutmeg spice. She felt an instant affinity, though she could not exactly say why. "Lady McKensie," she smiled. On impulse, she followed with, "Catherine, if you prefer." She liked this woman.

Flossie disappeared for a few minutes, and then returned with a tray of tea and a small plate of biscuits. She set the tray on the turned wood table, then poured the steaming liquid into a cup and set it before Catherine.

Catherine took a sip, and closed her eyes, feeling the hot liquid burn her throat. The pungent brew warmed her chilled insides. She set the cup back on the table. "Are you new to the village? I've not seen you before."

"I am, indeed, Milady. I came from London just before the plague took hold."

Catherine admired the woman's straightforward manner. "How did you happen to settle in our small village?"

Flossie glanced down the hall where the rowdy shouts of laughter had subsided into quiet murmurings. She seemed unsure of her manners with an aristocrat. Catherine gave her an encouraging smile and gestured to a chair. Flossie hesitated, taking the measure of the curious young woman sitting before her. Relenting, Flossie perched on the edge of the chair, as though ready to flee back to the public room should anyone call out. "T'was a man I met in London—an' a right fine man, 'e was, indeed. Just signed his son to a sailin' ship at the docks across from the Ratcliff Inn where I worked for a time..."

The Ratcliff Inn. Where had she heard the name before?

"...The gentleman didna' look like one of the regulars, though, and right as rain, 'e only wanted a pint an' a quiet moment of contemplations for the course he 'ad just set his son upon. Well, the plague had just come upon us all, an' 'e told me I should leave the city." Flossie idly scraped a drop of wax from the table with her fingernail. "I didna' have nowhere's to go, though. I 'ad no money, either..."

T'was MaryPryde... MaryPryde once worked at the inn.

...Flossie leaned over the table toward Catherine, speaking in confidence. "Well, d'ye know, the gentleman gave me four gold crowns right there and then, an' told me I might find employment in Wells. At the coaching inn. An' 'e was right. They gave me a position the very day I got off the coach from the north, an' I've been here since." She paused a moment, remembering the encounter. "Lord Abbott from Stockbridge, was 'is name."

Catherine smiled softly. The woman's praises were nothing new to the daughter of Sir Alvyn Abbott.

"Did ye know of him? Ay'n t'was a lamentable agony indeed to hear he had passed o' the plague."

Catherine hesitated a moment as the familiar ache returned. "He was my father," she whispered.

Flossie's eyes grew soft. Looking as though she wished to hug Catherine, Flossie instead turned her gaze toward the planked floor made pale in the soft winter light. She picked at a piece of lint on her sleeve. "'E changed my life, Lady Catherine," she whispered. "An' 'tis forever grateful, I'll be."

The noise from the public room faded as the two women sat in silence, thinking of the extraordinary man that meant so much to them both. Catherine looked out the window once more. The snow had stopped and the sun peeked through the heavy clouds that hung over the valley. After a few moments, Catherine stood, putting on her gloves.

"Yer leavin'? I 'aven't upset ye, nae, 'ave I?" asked Flossie, quickly rising from the chair in alarm.

Catherine caught Flossie's hands into her own, her dark gray eyes sparkling with tears. "No, Flossie, you have not caused an upset." They walked arm in arm toward the door. "Your story has touched me, indeed." She wiped her eyes. "He was a remarkable man. I was privileged to be his daughter." At that, Flossie's own eyes filled with sympathetic tears.

"Hello? Hello?" called a woman from the hallway, interrupting the moment. "Where is everyone?" she demanded.

Flossie immediately composed herself and ran out to the hallway. "Right 'ere, Lady Houghton, 'tis right 'ere that I am," she called out, flustered.

The woman swept into the private room, removing her gloves. "There is but an hour before the London coach departs and I should like to have tea before..." Lady Houghton stopped, staring at Catherine in surprise. Neither woman spoke. Lady Houghton gave Catherine a critical look from head to toe, and then broke the awkward silence.

"Hello, my dear," she said, brushing past Catherine toward a table by the window. She sat, taking moment to compose herself, and then turned to address Catherine.

"I see that congratulations are in order," she said, getting straight to the point.

Catherine absently twisted the ring on her finger. "Thank you, Lady Houghton. You and your family are well, I hope?" Catherine hesitated. "How is Miles?"

Lady Houghton waited a moment before speaking. "Still in France," she said, gazing at Catherine, her distain palpable. "I had hoped he would return for the Christmas Ball in two weeks time, although I don't know if he can bear it, such was his humiliation at your hand."

If he is in need of funds to pay his gambling debts, Miles will indeed return like a trick farthing. Catherine shifted, uncomfortably. "My apologies, I...I thought ending the engagement was for the best for all concerned, Lady Hough..."

Lady Houghton cut her off. "I fear an invitation was not sent to the Abbey this year. I presumed you and your family would be in London," she sniffed. "You understand, of course."

Catherine straightened her spine. *How grateful I am to have escaped this woman's clutches.* "Please do not trouble yourself over the invitation, Lady Houghton." Catherine stepped back, bowing her head in polite deference to the older woman as she retreated. "We are not quite in the festive spirit this year." As the older woman digested the rebuke, Catherine nodded once more, and then walked out the door.

Flossie followed close behind, helping Catherine retrieve her cloak from the peg in the hallway.

"The Lady Houghton can be a bit demanding. I hope she has not frightened you off?"

"I know her well, Flossie. She does not frighten me." She fastened the closures of her cloak, and then set her hand to Flossie's arm. "I'm glad you've come to the village. Toby is very fond of you," she smiled. "I shall come back soon, I promise."

As Catherine left, shouts from the public room took Flossie back to her duties. Catherine stepped outside and waited while Toby brought her horse. Lifting her by the knee into the saddle, he watched as Catherine clicked her teeth and turned the horse down hill toward the deserted stable yards.

"Careful, Lady Catherine," he called out. "No one goes near the stables anymore."

Catherine nodded in agreement. *She had no intention of riding into the stableyard.* The wrenching memories were still far too fresh. Giving the burned out building a very wide berth, Catherine rode to a deserted field behind the rolling pasturelands. As she trotted around a hedgerow she caught her breath and pulled the horse up sharply at the sight of thirteen simple wooden crosses fronting the pasture where Simon had buried the plague victims. She had fallen from a tree once when she was young, and the sharp blow to her back made her feel as though the air had been knocked from her body. Lying motionless on the ground, she truly felt in those terror-stricken moments that she might die. Seeing the graves for the first time since the quarantine made her feel exactly the same as she had lying beneath the oak tree. *She felt as though she couldn't breathe.*

Barely able to look upon the sight of the crosses, she moved down the row, forcing herself to count to nine, and then dismounted. Tears filled her eyes. She leaned back against the horse, desolate in her sorrow, somber in the contemplation of her father's grave. Her knees felt weak. *T'was near incomprehensible that he this day lay quiet in the earth.* She leaned down and ran her hand over the snow-dusted mound. *How could she ever have left him there alone? How could she leave him all alone now?* The horse, as if sensing her pain, whinnied and nuzzled her cheek. She gazed upon her father's grave. *The stillness, the stark finality of it all was impossible to comprehend.* Clutching the reins, Catherine finally broke down into heart-breaking, guttural sobs, unable to contain the grief that overwhelmed.

The afternoon sun broke through the clouds once more. Ice crystals glinted across the wind-swept fields. Catherine marveled at the sparkling landscape and collected herself, her grief spent. She dried her tears and then stood, a fragile acceptance slowly quelling her sorrow. She walked a short distance into the woods, brushing through the fragrant pine branches and chokecherry shrubs in her path. Breaking off several hawthorn branches laden with bright red berries, she fashioned the stems into a makeshift bouquet, then tied the branches together with a ribbon from her hair. She paused a moment and closed her eyes. A robin's trill echoed across the silent pasture. She felt an icy breeze across her face as it rustled through the pines boughs. *'Tis a beautiful resting spot, indeed.* A sudden, riotous chirping cut short her moment of contemplation. Catherine opened her eyes wide to a frenzied clutch of finches attacking the berries, the birds made drunk and unsteady from the intoxicating nectar. She burst into unexpected laughter, and then shook the bouquet to scatter the birds away. Catherine turned and walked back toward the fence. She laid the bouquet atop her father's grave, the bright red berries a stark contrast to the white snow. She stood alone over the slight rise in the ground and sighed, still not quite believing it all had happened.

"Catherine!"

She whirled around to see Simon on horseback racing down the hill, his cloak billowing behind him.

"Catherine!" he called out again.

"What is it?" she cried, reaching up for the bridle as he drew close.

"The Lord Mayor has been taken with the fevers." He dismounted and took her into his arms. "He will live, Catherine. The mayor will live."

CHAPTER TWENTY-SEVEN

Abbottsford Abbey
Stockbridge, Buckinghamshire
3 January 1667

Catherine wandered through the quiet abbey, waiting for Simon to examine the mayor one last time before they left for London. Gazing at the timbered entrance hall, as if to memorize every last inch of the home she loved, her eyes fell upon the painting Viola had insisted they save from Bealeton House. It had been propped against the back wall awaiting its eventual return to London. She caught her breath. It was as though her father stood before her once more. Not for the first time did she think he would have loved to have spent more time with Simon, for the two were kindred souls in so many ways.

The holidays had come and gone quietly. Though the mayor had been permitted an hour from his bedside to join in a round of basset on Christmas Day, and although the card game was merry, they all felt the overwhelming undercurrent of sadness, for the day was strange and melancholy without Sir Abbott. Simon had given her a new illustration quill with a golden, filigreed hilt, touching her once again with his thoughtfulness. Without time to visit the shops while helping Viola care for the mayor, Catherine had wrapped a treasured book and set it upon the stone hearth in the gathering room where a simple Yule log burned. Simon had seemed pleased with the copy of John Milton's poems, though she could not be entirely sure that poetry was a favored subject of his. With her father's death and the mayor's illness, they all felt keenly the emptiness of the holiday season.

By the first of January, the fevers had well run their course, and the mayor was recovering apace. They had spent nearly a month at the Abbey, giving Catherine time enough to finish detailing the front, back and side drawings of Berkshire House for Lady Wilbraham, well in advance of the mid-March deadline. Though Simon and Charles had travelled to London each week since the fevers had first come upon the mayor, returning only at the weekends, after such a lengthy interval Simon was more than anxious to return to the hospital full time. Charles, deep into his first year studies, was ready to return to his Lincoln's Inn dormitory as well. The mayor had chuffed vociferously at what seemed to him an endless confinement, but, in an abundance of caution, Simon had ordered another three months rest before he and Viola could even contemplate a return to London. Viola had stamped her dainty foot down to Cecil's most vocal objections and that, thought Catherine with amusement, had been that.

The doorway to the library was slightly ajar. Catherine hesitated a moment with her hand on the doorknob, and then, steeling herself, pushed the door open and walked in. *It was as though time itself had stopped.* Sir Abbott's papers and books lay opened exactly as he had left them. His maps were spread across a wide library table in his dogged quest to find more economical trade routes to India and the Far East. His spectacles lay untouched atop his papers. Even the familiar, comforting scent of his pipe tobacco clung still to the books and the thick tapestry window coverings. A blue and cream-colored Delftware jar filled with hard spun sugar candies sat on the desk. She lifted the lid and inhaled, then closed her eyes, instantly lost in a swirl of wistful memories, for she and her father alone shared a love of the sweet, sticky barley twists.

She set the lid back, suddenly struck by the oddest of feelings. The sensation persisted as she ran her fingers across the rough parchments on his writing table. Although she had stood at the foot of his grave and was under no fanciful illusions, it somehow felt as if the newness of her father's death had worn off and she was now left with the thought that he had somehow simply gone away and would return at any moment, filling the house once more with his merry humor and wise counsel. Yet she knew he would not return. *He would never return.* Though the feeling saddened her in full measure, at this moment, she felt strangely, inexplicably emboldened. In his quiet, determined way, Sir Abbott had raised his children with the courage to chart their own course. She now knew that she possessed strength enough to make her own decisions. The realization struck her like a thunderbolt. *She no longer needed to hear his words, for they were forever imprinted in her heart.* She *knew* what to do. She stood alone in the library for several long minutes absorbing the enormity of that thought and then, finally finding herself at peace, Catherine turned and walked from the library, quietly closing the door behind her.

Back in the entrance hall, she took her traveling hat from a table beneath a gilded mirror. Through a leaded glass window by the entry door, she caught a glimpse of Jock loading their bags atop the carriage. He bent down and grabbed another case, then hoisted it high. A sudden movement made him turn abruptly. Grinning, Jock sank to a knee and held his arms held out. Catherine shifted her gaze to see the kitchen maid, Annie, bent over, holding the tiny fingers of a little tow-headed girl toddling through the snow. Catherine dropped the hat and ran out to the courtyard.

"She's walking, Annie!" Catherine cried out.

"Aye, Milady, she is indeed," laughed Annie, her eyes shining.

Catherine swung the little girl up into her arms and hugged her tightly, jouncing from foot to foot. "Such a sweet little moppet, your Elsbeth is!" Catherine tickled the little girl under the chin, and then swept her hand across the unruly blond curls that tumbled down her forehead. "Miss Elsbeth Catherine." The little girl looked up at Catherine, giggling and cooing. A translucent spit bubble popped on her tiny, bow-shaped lips. Elsbeth giggled again.

"We're forever thankful to ye, Milady, for savin' Annie's life," said Jock, wrapping his arms around Annie.

"Aye, Milady, 'tis grateful we are, indeed" said Annie, bowing her head in gratitude.

Catherine smiled, handing Elsbeth back to her mother. "I am only too glad that I was there that night and was able to help." Elsbeth giggled and reached out for Catherine, her chubby fingers opening and closing in playful teasings. To the little girl's delight Catherine put her hands over her eyes, playing *pique-a-boo*.

"Soon ye'll be havin' wee ones of yer own," laughed Annie. Jock looked at her sharply. Annie stepped back and bowed her head. "My apologies, Milady, I...I spoke out of turn," she murmured. Elsbeth gave a little cry of outrage, bouncing impatiently in her mother's arms.

"Aye, that would be lovely indeed, Annie," reassured Catherine, playfully hiding her eyes once more. Elsbeth kicked her feet out and squealed in glee.

The front door opened. Viola walked arm in arm with Charles out to the carriage. Simon followed, carrying Catherine's small travel case. He set it inside the coach, and then turned back to Viola. "Allow the mayor one hour of amusement each day, but persuade him to stay abed as much as possible," he instructed.

"He'll not listen to me long, I fear."

Simon laughed. "Nae, I do not think he will, either. But rest assured, Lady Viola, that in itself is a very good sign, indeed."

Upstairs, a window sash was thrown wide. The mayor poked his head through the opening and shook his fist down to an unrepentant Simon. "I'll not stay in that infernal bed one single moment longer than you require, laddie!" he cried out. The mayor ducked his head back inside before Simon could raise an objection and slammed the window shut.

Simon grinned at Viola. "'Tis quite a long confinement you have ahead, Lady Hardwicke." At that, Simon, Catherine, and Charles boarded the rig and settled in for the ride back to London. The coach pulled away. Simon leaned out of the carriage window. "Long confinement, indeed."

"Drive on, Mr. Fitch!" called Viola, laughing as she waved them away. "Drive on…" Viola stood alone, watching as the carriage disappeared down the snowy lane.

CHAPTER TWENTY-EIGHT

"NO GREAT DISCOVERY WAS EVER MADE
WITHOUT FIRST A BOLD GUESS"
~ SIR ISAAC NEWTON

St. Bartholomew's Hospital
Smithfield Parish, London
3 March 1667

Again, sir? You...you wish to do what?" spluttered a bewhiskered man as he stood before Simon dressed in clothes once fine, now tattered and ragged. The man dared a quick glance through the nearby window as if to plot an urgent escape. The sight of the melting snows that had been piled as high as a horse's chest made him pull his cloak tighter, though he could not say entirely whether he was chilled, or rather that he felt he needed the protection. An eerie, howling wind whistling through the timbers above lent a particularly ominous note to the unthinkable enterprise. The man stared down at a leaflet that had been thrust into his hands by a young boy outside the hospital. His jaw hung slack with disbelief. He held the paper out to the length of his arm and squinted at the text once more.

Sitting behind a desk, Simon took hold of the notes he had compiled from the Oxford research and for the eleventh time that morning, read aloud the intended course, ticking off each point. "The day before the experiment, you will be admitted into the hospital, given a hot meal and a clean bed. You will also be given a full medical examination from head to foot before you retire for the night. The following morning, you will take your place in the research theater where you will be the subject of a blood transfusion experiment."

Incredulous, the man stared down at the gruesome illustrations Simon had spread across the table. He took a wary step backward.

"While you are on the table, Father Hardwicke, the medical students and I will examine you once more," Simon continued, concentrating on his notes. "Then, I will take a scissure in your right arm and your blood will be let. After an interval, we will take the measure of that blood. In your left arm, another scissure will be taken. One end of a goose quill will be inserted into the cleft of the second scissure. At the other end of the quill, a sheep's bladder filled with sheep's blood will drip that blood through the quill into your arm in such equal quantity as to the blood that was let. We will then keep close watch on you and document the results as they appear. For your service we offer three gold cr…"

Simon looked up sharply at the sound of the parchment hitting the floor. He watched in dismay as the man charged through the great hall toward the doorway, then leaned his elbows on the desk and sighed. Running his fingers through his hair in frustration, Simon looked out across the teeming hall and waved to the leaflet boy once more.

CHAPTER TWENTY-NINE

Wilbraham Manor
St. James Place, London
3 March 1667

ady Wilbraham led Catherine down a wide, planked hallway lined with flickering candle sconces and muted woolen carpets to a doorway with an intriguing, engraved doorlatch. Catherine stopped a moment to admire the ornamented craftsmanship of the forged-iron latch and the tulip-shaped strap hinges that secured the door to the frame. The attention to detail in the Wilbraham mansion was breathtaking.

"This way, Catherine," smiled Elizabeth, opening the door. She saw Catherine's interest and pointed to the tulip hinges as they passed through the entry. "The flower of the Netherlands. I once spent a great deal of time there," she said, modest in her architectural education.

Catherine caught her breath. Though not as grand in scale as the larger public rooms, the room was magnificent. The outside walls of the book-filled chamber were lined with soaring arched windows, flooding the chamber with light, even in the snowy, winter gloom. Richly patterned rugs from India and the Near East warmed the planked floor. A collection of exotic, flowering orchids in clay pots lined the wide sills, bright spots of crimson and coral against the gray afternoon skies. Several candelabras were spaced evenly around a large table, casting a warm light upon stacks of papers and an ordered collection of inkpots and drawing instruments. A second, smaller table was illuminated by three more candlestands, one on each side and one at the back. The smaller tabletop was slanted upwards at the rear. A young candle boy finished lighting the wicks and hurried from the room.

"My drawing office," said Elizabeth, gesturing wide.

Catherine walked to the angled table and looked carefully at its construction. She set her fingertips to the iron rods that lifted the drawing board and then upon the slim piece of wood at the base that kept papers and drawing instruments from sliding off. "'Tis curious."

"A tilted drawing table. Have you not seen one?"

Catherine shook her head. "Nae, I have not. Why is it tilted upwards?"

"An excellent question, as they are unusual, indeed. Tilting the drawing board accommodates the eyes visual perception of perspective and foreshortening. You perhaps encountered this the first time you drew a column? There is a tendency towards an exaggerated perspective in the vertical direction, which if not accommodated, usually results in the capstone appearing too tall."

"A puzzlement solved!" Catherine mused. "I did, in fact, make several corrections on my first attempt, but I did not understand why the proportions seemed off." Catherine reached into her valise. "Perhaps I might raise my own desk on books to achieve the same result?" she wondered, handing over a stack of papers. "Here are the finished drawings for Berkshire House."

Elizabeth spread the papers across the larger table, and nodded her approval. "These views, the front, back and side views of the house are called elevations, and you have completed them beautifully. Your drawings will complement my specifications well. Will you allow me to compensate you for your time?"

"Please do not think of it, Elizabeth. My uncle has been quite ill in Stockbridge and we have been looking after him during his recuperation. I was grateful for something to do." Catherine looked once more at the worktable. "If I may, specifications?" she asked. "I apologize, but the terms are unfamiliar."

Elizabeth pointed to a thick, loosely bound sheaf of papers at the side of the table. "The structural specifications." Catherine furrowed her brow, still not quite understanding. "These are the plans for the foundation, the vaults, the domes, the roof—the entire project," Elizabeth explained. "Every single element of the design—from the exact cost and amount of the materials ordered, to the strength and placement of everything from the base layer to the roof trusses, to the landscape design and planting instructions—must be described in exact detail so that the contractor and the craftsmen are able to construct the building. Your work, along with the specifications, will aid in conveying that information."

"I had no idea," marveled Catherine, her appreciation growing tenfold for the effort Viola had put into Bealeton House. Catherine picked up an unusual drawing instrument from a wooden box. "May I ask what this is?"

"It's called a reservoir pen." Elizabeth took the pen from Catherine and pointed to a wide barrel above the nib. "My husband purchased it in Germany on our wedding trip. You see the pen is made from two quills." She held it out for Catherine to examine. "One quill is placed inside the other and the ink goes in the reservoir, which is closed with a cork." She pulled the small cork. Catherine looked inside. "The ink flows from the center quill through a small hole down to the nib. I find it excellent for shading."

"Fascinating," Catherine murmured. "Your husband is very thoughtful."

Elizabeth paused a moment. "He was very thoughtful, indeed."

Catherine looked up, questioning, as she handed the quill back to Elizabeth.

"I am six years a widow, Catherine," said Elizabeth, returning the quill to its box. "Financially, I am well cared for as my husband was much older than I, but when he died, I was 29 years old. I…I found myself wandering the house with no purpose. I spent weeks, months even, yearning for what I had lost and pining for my husband terribly. He believed in my talents, going so far as to extend our wedding trip six years so that I could study architecture abroad. After he died, I was very sad and the days were very long. But I had designed our country home, and an opportunity from friends presented another project, which led to one more after that, and now, here I am," she smiled.

"I am truly sorry," said Catherine. "I, too, have lost someone very dear to me." They fell silent for a moment, each contemplating the aching loss of someone they loved.

"Life does have a way of moving forward," said Elizabeth, brightening the conversation. "How did you and your husband meet? A physick, is he not? I might think it a very different story from the customary social arrangements."

"Yes, Simon is a physick at St. Bartholomew's. He was sent to our village of Wells to care for the Lord Mayor, and when the plague came to us, Simon treated the sick very differently than they were treated here in London. He used an experimental method of isolation, and because of that isolation, only thirteen perished. I helped him with the research that will become his second book."

"He has published a book, as well?"

"Yes, on both blood circulation and medical practices on the spread of disease."

"I shall have to purchase this book by Dr. Simon McKensie."

"You will find it under the name of Dr. Robert Marlowe. He used a *nom de plume,* as he was unsure of using his own name while in medical training. He will use his own name on his second book.

"Dr. Robert Marlowe as a *nom de plume.* How terribly accomplished your husband is." Elizabeth smiled. "I believe you were meant for each other."

Catherine blushed, nodding in agreement. "Whatever I have achieved pales in comparison." She turned to Elizabeth, daring to express a troubling thought in the unguarded moment.

"You, yourself, are quite accomplished, Lady…Elizabeth. May I ask—the other women I met, are they equally so? I fear I may not 'measure up.'"

Elizabeth laughed, a girlish peal that delighted Catherine. "Each in their own way, yes. I believe we found one another for that very reason, and there is no reason to fear. You 'measure up' quite well. We enjoy your company very much, Catherine."

Catherine blushed. "Thank you, I feel the same."

Elizabeth turned thoughtful. "Bathsua is by far the most learned of us all. She was the tutor to Elizabeth Stuart, the daughter of King Charles I. She is fluent in Greek, Latin, Hebrew, German, Spanish, French and Italian, and has written several treatises championing the equal right of women to obtain an education. In fact, she intends one day to find a willing investor and open a school for young, impoverished girls. Eight years a widow with little inheritance, she must needs provide for herself, and she has done so, with great effort and intelligent resourcefulness. Bathsua is violently opposed to the prevailing thought of woman as the weaker vessels, subordinated to man and uneducable," Elizabeth smiled, "and she makes her opinions very well known."

Catherine thought of MaryPryde and the cruel way she had been treated by her husband. "I quite agree with her," said Catherine, grateful that MaryPryde was free of the despicable man.

"Dear Aphra earns her living by writing plays and fictional novels, a first for a woman in England," Elizabeth leaned in close, "and although she will not speak of it, she has just returned from Antwerp where she has obtained, shall we say, certain information for the King." She sifted through the collection of parchment papers, examining Catherine's work once more. "Though the King has been rather slow to recompense," confided Elizabeth, arching an eyebrow. "Perhaps he feels that a woman has no need of an income, but that which is provided by a husband. Aphra is two years a widow, but she was left without funds, save that which she provides for *herself*."

"Espionage in service to the King? She appears quite fragile," said Catherine, impulsively. She ducked her head and vowed once more to refrain from expressing her thoughts in such a direct fashion.

"Ahh, but do not let appearances fool you, Catherine. Our perceived fragility is often our greatest strength."

"My own mother had that quality," said Catherine, chagrined. "She was often underestimated."

"And Pippa, our darling Pippa, is quite the entrancing and entertaining hostess. Capable of laying a generous table of such artistry that astounds even the most staid and sober of guests. One is grateful for an invitation to even a single gathering she gets up. That sharp wit and keen intelligence of hers attracts all manner of admirers to her orbit, including The Countess of Castlemaine, the king's mistress."

Catherine's eyes widened at the mention of a mistress to the King, but this time, she kept her tongue.

"I told you we stand on no ceremony here, Catherine," laughed Elizabeth, as she set her hands upon the stack of specifications. "Berkshire House is the king's gift to the countess. I consider myself very fortunate to have his faith and trust in my work." She gave Catherine a curious glance. "Perhaps you would like to meet her? The countess holds a salon in her quarters nearly every night. The other ladies rarely attend, but Pippa is drawn to the gaming tables, while I must keep myself in the king's good graces for the work. Men are included to share cigars and brandy in the king's company. Have you and your husband been presented at court?"

"Although I have no memory of the occasion, I was once presented to his father, King Charles I, at a ball my father gave when I was very young, but, no, I have not had the honor."

Elizabeth, warming to the idea, took Catherine's hands into her own. "If you will not allow me to compensate you for your time, you must let me arrange an introduction. There is a gathering in two nights time, you must come!"

"I'm afraid my husband may not take to the idea. He is not one for parties," she paused, "although it does sound lovely."

"Perhaps he would make an exception this once?"

Catherine looked over to the desk filled with architectural plans created by Elizabeth. She marveled at these accomplished, intelligent and very resourceful women. Women who had the respect of the king. Women who had the respect of their husbands as equals. Women who had purpose and did exactly as they wished to do. *She wanted to be a part of their world.* "Perhaps he would."

CHAPTER THIRTY

Whitehall Palace
Westminster, Middlesex,
London, England
Saturday, 5 March 1667

"She is a married man!" hissed Simon, as they waited in an interminable carriage line approaching Whitehall Palace. "I do not understand why it is you wish an introduction to his "mistress," or to socialize with those who would condone such a dishonorable practice." Simon shifted his muscular frame uncomfortably in a slightly small, yet fashionable court costume. "The Merry Monarch, my foot," he grumbled. The deep red velvet waistcoat and black beribboned formal breeches borrowed from Charles restricted his movements across the back and added to his irritation. Jutting his jaw forward, he pulled at the cravat wound tightly around his neck for some measure of relief. "I do not understand the ways of aristocrats. What's more, I feel perfectly ridiculous in this periwig," he said, swiping at the curls that tickled his neck.

He watched as Catherine shot a quick glance up toward Fitch who, sitting on the bench outside, was guiding the horses through the narrow West End lanes. Satisfied that the driver could not hear their exchange, she turned toward Simon seemingly unfazed by his momentary display of ill humor. She spoke gently. "I do not judge the King, nor do I wish to condemn when I do not entirely know the facts—except to say that I, too, was once the unwitting subject of an arranged marriage."

Simon fell silent, brought up short by her mention of the man he considered a cowardly fool. He played with the garter on Charles' breeches, laying first the ribbon on one side of his leg, and then shifting the ties to the other. "Nothing looks right. Ridiculous embellishment," he murmured.

"Imagine being forced by ministers of the crown to marry a woman unknown to you simply for the financial benefit of the monarchy, as I was once nearly forced to marry Miles Houghton for the financial and social benefit of my aunt? I would have sympathy for each actor in a play were such a play produced, and I believe you would too—were you not quite so prejudiced against those with whom you are unfamiliar," she said in a soft, yet impassioned whisper.

The fizz withered from his bluster. He had been out of sorts for weeks and although he had tried to hide it, the frustrating delay of his experiment was causing him nothing but vexation. Simon contemplated the ribbons he held, berating himself for his vexations, then dropped them and turned to her. "No, I cannot imagine being held to such a scheme. You are right, Catherine," he said, chagrined. The carriage moved forward toward the gothic arched entrance, then stopped once more. "My apologies. I have no right to judge, as I am indeed, quite unfamiliar with your world. The differences in our upbringing has not mattered in the least, yet, in this moment, I wish no more than to return to Bealeton House, for I fear I will have nothing in common and nothing to speak of with the other guests," he confessed, in a rare moment of doubt.

"There are few as intelligent and accomplished as you, Simon. Anyone this night would consider themselves fortunate to spend time with you. I foremost among them," she smiled.

Much relieved, Simon set his hand upon hers and gave it a slight squeeze. Pulling her close, the soft scent of Gussie's thyme soap delighted his senses. He looked at her red hair set off by a cloak of dark green wool and the earbobs of emerald stones that peeked from its fur-lined hood. *How is it possible that on this night, she is even more beautiful?* She turned up to him smiling an incandescent smile that lifted his spirits and made his heart soar. He could not hold himself back. *Hang the gown and the arranged hair!* He drew her close and kissed her, a deep, longing kiss filled with the gratitude of one who had never been loved and grateful once more to the fates that brought them together.

"Any moment now, Milady!" yelled down Fitch, as he guided the horses toward the stone gatehouse arch that led to the palace entrance.

Laughing, Catherine pushed Simon's hands away, straightening her cloak and hair. "There will be time enough…" she scolded, playfully.

Simon stared through the glass at the palace as they drew closer. He wrinkled his brow in bewilderment. The central hall of the palace had been built in alternating layers of pink and honey-colored stone, highlighted by the white Portland stone that gave Whitehall its name, but the layout was irregular and its many side buildings were of different sizes and architectural styles. "Whitehall looks more like a small town rather than one single building. I would have thought a palace to have a certain, ah… grandeur. This looks to be a rather higglty-pigglty heap of houses." he mused.

Catherine glanced out to the riotous jumble of Tudor, Italian Renaissance and Jacobean buildings wedged around the perimeter of the massive royal grounds. "The palace does look rather unimpressive from the outside," murmured Catherine, "although as a child, I remember vividly the inside of the Banqueting Hall being very grand." She pulled the invitation from her black velvet handbag and looked down to the meticulous calligraphy, its swirling ascending and descending letters elaborate swoops on the parchment much like birds soaring in flight. "We are to be received in the Banqueting Hall, then we are invited to the countesses chambers for gaming and *bonne bouche.*"

Simon leaned his head back against the bench. Although he had no earthly idea what a *bonne bouche* was, he was certain he did not want one. The hollow sound of hooves clopping on the cobblestones echoed through the dim, narrow archway that led into the palace grounds. He closed his eyes and groaned as the horses picked up speed toward what surely promised to be an uncomfortable evening with no prospect of escape.

***

"Doctor and Lady Simon McKensie," cried a formally attired footman standing at the top of the marble steps that led down into the Banqueting Hall. With all the enthusiasm of a man headed to the gaol, Simon offered his arm, and he and Catherine ventured down into the reception area.

In one corner of the hall, a consort of lute players played variations by Purcell, to the delight of the fawning guests. Simon glanced up to the white painted walls and second floor side galleries in the vast, cavernous hall, but as he walked the length of the crimson and gold floral carpet, he could not look away from the spectacular ceiling. Walnut-tree stained and richly gilded in gold leaf, the partitioned ceiling was embellished with nine magnificent oils painted by the Flemish ar'tist, Peter Paul Reubens. Still craning his gaze upwards in awe of the jewel-toned paintings that glorified the achievements of the King's father, Charles I, Simon stumbled on the ruffle of Catherine's gown. He froze a moment, terrified that he might have damaged the fabric. Regaining his balance. Catherine gave him a sly, reassuring wink as they continued the long walk toward the King. "'Tis fine," she murmured.

At the far end of the carpet, in a gilded throne placed upon an elevated platform, sat King Charles II, resplendent in a billowing mass of royal blue satin robes. A thick, gold crown studded with emeralds and sapphires sat upon his luxurious brown periwig.

Deep in thought, he stared above the crowd, as though distracted and wholly uninterested in either the ceremony or the assembled guests. As the footman escorted Catherine and Simon forward, two small puppies broke free from their handler and bounded onto the platform, yipping incessantly as they darted to and fro between the white tights of the Monarch's legs. The King suddenly sprang to life, shouting in great merriment.

"Jollyboy! Lillups!" he cried, bending down to lift the excitable red and white spaniels into his lap. Delighting in the creatures, he held first one puppy aloft and then the other to the excitement of the crowd. After a few moments, he settled the dogs in his lap. He stroked their soft fur with long, thin, bejeweled fingers, and in the moment of calm, the king seemed to succumb once again to distraction and worry. He idly waved at the footman to continue.

"Doctor and Lady Simon McKensie!"

Paying no heed to the riotous disruption, Catherine set one foot behind the other and curtsied low. She spoke quietly. "Your Majesty."

Though thoroughly ill at ease, Simon, as Catherine had instructed, bowed deeply at the waist. He lifted his head. "Your Royal Highness," he said, in a clear speaking voice, with far more bravado than he felt.

Fondling the puppy's ears, the king nodded in vague acknowledgment. The curious spaniels pulled from his grasp and clambered up the king's sash, licking at his cheeks and razor-thin mustache as the crowd cheered once more. In the midst of the frivolity, Catherine felt oddly as though the king's glance had lingered upon her a moment longer than custom would allow. Simon seemed nothing but grateful that the encounter was over and heaved a great sigh that no disaster had befallen them. From there the footman led them to one side, then disappeared to escort the remaining guests down the carpet. Catherine and Simon were left alone in the crowd.

"Lady McKensie!" Catherine turned to see Elizabeth approaching through the mass of courtesans and courtiers. She was dressed in an exquisite gown of pale gold taffeta and ivory lace, embellished by an unusual, languid twist of charcoal satin that draped low across the back of the skirt. "I've been watching for you."

"Eliz…Lady Wilbraham," said Catherine, catching herself. She set her hand on Simon's arm. "May I present my husband, Simon McKensie."

"Lady Wilbraham," nodded Simon, quite aware that the less said, the less one might put one's foot in it.

"'Tis a pleasure to make your acquaintance, sir," said Elizabeth. She winked at Catherine as she placed her hand through the crook of Simon's arm. "Come with me, Doctor," she said, her eyes sparkling. "I have the feeling that a large gathering such as this is not entirely to your taste."

∾⚬∾

Icy snow drifted through a series of open-air stone arches as the threesome walked along a balcony above the palace's interior courtyard. Snowflakes collected in the fur of Catherine's hood, clinging to her eyelashes and cheeks. Walking the balcony's length in the soft torchlight, they at last came upon a doorway to the private apartments. Shouts of laughter and excitable conversation could be heard from the illuminated crack beneath the door. Simon hung back, looking quite uncomfortable. Elizabeth reached for the gold knocker and dropped it once against the backplate. Moments later, another footman in formal attire swung the door wide, smiling in welcome.

"Welcome, Milord, Miladies," he intoned, ushering them inside the fire-warmed entrance hall. A uniformed maid standing to one side offered them each a shallow champagne coupe filled with sparkling Blanquette de Limoux from a silver tray.

Simon accepted a glass and followed as the footman escorted them into the expansive gathering room. He took a sip and then froze, his glass suspended in mid-air as he gaped, open-mouthed at the sheer opulence that lay before him. Had he not felt so out of place among the extravagantly dressed courtiers and courtesans, he might have laughed aloud at the pink and gold embellishments that filled the room.

The walls were covered in a folly of hand-stenciled murals. Gold-leafed angels peeked from billowing clouds on a pink milk-painted background. Gold candle chandeliers that hung from the ceiling dripped with cascading crystal bobs, as did the golden wall sconces. The furnishings were softened with pillows in every shade of pink velvet. Rose-colored carpets covered the pale oak floorings. The crowning touch at the center of the room was a pink marble statue of cupid kneeling on a rock, shooting a stream of water from his bow. Simon was incredulous. He had a difficult time keeping a straight face as he took another sip of champagne. He fought to keep it down.

"Lady Wilbraham! Lady McKensie!" cried a voice from the gaming tables arranged at the back of the room. "Your appearance could not be more well timed," she called out. The dark-haired woman in a low-cut, black silk gown threw her cards to the table in surrender, then arose from her chair and rushed toward them, arms outstretched. A voluptuous chestnut-haired woman on the opposite side of the table stacked the coins left behind with a merry laugh. A coterie of giggling courtesans applauded her efforts.

"Lady Phillipa Dillworth," murmured Catherine.

Simon saw the lively Lady Dillworth approaching, enthusiastic in her intended charge. Wary and uncomfortable, he retreated a step. *Something is wrong.* He glanced to his left and right. The room was full of women. *Not one man in sight.* An impending dread began to rise in his chest. He had never felt so out of place in his life. Elizabeth excused herself to greet the countess at the games table. Pippa, taking Catherine and Simon well in hand, escorted them around the room with introductions to so many women his head began to ache. Finally, witness to his discomfort, she stopped.

"I believe you have reached a limit, sir," Pippa smiled. She glanced back to the chestnut-haired woman who was intently gazing at her hand of cards. "You shall meet the countess after our *bonne bouche.* In the meantime, I think you might feel a bit more comfortable in the company of men." She turned to a courtesan standing nearby. "Perhaps you would entertain Lady McKensie for a moment? She might enjoy watching the game." The girl gave a warm smile and led Catherine to the tables. Pippa took Simon by the crook of his arm with a playful tug. "We shall return." As she led him through an arched opening into another chamber, Simon looked back to Catherine, his eyes begging for reprieve.

Simon followed Pippa into a small library, this chamber far more masculine in decoration than the last. Hand-tooled leather chairs were arranged in small groupings before a soaring paneled mantelpiece. Men clustered around the fire, chatting amiably over tots of brandy. Others were seated at the heavy wooden game tables, each to a man shouting in vigorous competition. Though the atmosphere suited him far more than the pink angels, once again, Simon felt very ill at ease.

"Lady Dillworth!" cried an excitable voice. A slight young man dressed in the latest of fashionable formal attire ran toward them, carrying a bottle of champagne in one hand and a glass in the other. Two other equally high-spirited young men followed him closely. Simon could feel the instant tension as Pippa straightened her spine and turned to face them.

"I believe I have not had the pleasure of making this man's acquaintance," the young man cried, gleefully pouring more of the sparkling wine into his nearly full glass. Champagne sloshed over the rim of his glass. He winked at Simon and slowly licked the back of his hand.

Simon flinched at the uncomfortable display. Lifting her chin, Pippa smiled stiffly, her manners impeccable. "May I introduce Sir John Wilmot, the Second Earl of Rochester? And this is Mr. Baptist May, and Mr. Henry Killigrew, head of the King's Company theatricals. Gentlemen, I present the physick, Simon McKensie."

"Sir Wilmot, Mr. May and Mr. Killigrew." Simon nodded. He took in Wilmot's bleary eyes, his shaking hands and his unsteady gait.

"Aren't you quite the dashing one?" murmured Wilmot, tripping slightly over the edge of the carpet. "I do believe the king should enjoy meeting you this night…" He turned his head toward Killigrew, setting his hand aside his thin, delicate lips, "…if he weren't embroiled in another pique with the countess over your delicious Gwyn woman," he said, with a giddy wave of his fingertips toward the women's gaming tables. He set his arm around Simon's shoulder. "A low-born orange peddler in the stalls to the lead actress in the King's Company theatricals in less than a year—quite the leap, would you not say, Doctor?"

Simon removed Wilmot's arm and stepped away. "I am unfamiliar with theater gossip, sir."

Killigrew lifted an eyebrow. "She is quite the willing comic talent," he said, dryly.

Baptist May took a sip of champagne and leaned in with a conspiratorial whisper. "I have heard it well said that the king will not attend tonight's salon—he has gone into hiding." He glanced through the wide doorway toward the countess enthusiastically throwing coins to the table. "The capricious 'tides of temper' do not favor His Majesty at present."

"No!" pouted Wilmot, pouring more champagne. "My cards have been most excellent. I would have reveled in pillaging the king's purse. Or, at the very least, recoup a bit of my own, shall we say, rather considerable losses."

"His Majesty has this hour departed for Malmesbury House, and does not intend to return to London for at least a fortnight, perhaps longer, until…shall we say, the 'tides' turn," grinned

May, belaying a strong measure of enjoyment at sharing the tidbit of juicy gossip.

"He may have to stay in seclusion much longer than anticipated. She will not forgive easily," predicted Killigrew, holding his glass toward Wilmot. "He may also have to dangle another emerald necklace…"

"With the earbobs to match!" cried Wilmot, gleefully filling Killigrew's glass to the brim. Wilmot leaned in and nodded toward the countess. "I pity the messenger…"

Killigrew looked toward the high-spirited duchess playing in the gathering room. "A three-days ride is not nearly far enough to escape the wrath, if you ask me," he murmured under his breath. His eyes widened with interest. "Who is that delicious maid in green standing behind the countess? The one with the red hair? I do not believe I have well laid eyes upon her before this night."

"The king does favor red hair," smirked May. "Perhaps *she* could be enticed to "the theater." All three men laughed at the bawdy insinuation.

With a start, Simon realized they were speaking of Catherine. *There is no end to the deviltry!* Struck with a sudden fury at the ill-mannered implication, he drew himself to his full height, towering over the trio. "That gentlemen, is my *wife*," he said, through clenched teeth.

"Apologize this instant, Mr. May," demanded Pippa under her breath, her irritation at the threesome more than apparent.

"And a lovely woman she is, indeed. I beg your forgiveness, sir," said May, with a formal nod. Wilmot put his fingers to his lips to hide an unrepentant grin.

Simon calmed himself. "Aye, Mr. May, I accept your apology," he said, though not entirely convinced of the sincerity of May's repentance.

Wilmot shot Simon a sidelong glance from head to toe. "And you, sir? While the cat's away…," he purred.

"That is quite enough, Sir Wilmot," cautioned Pippa.

Wilmot let out a high-pitched giggle and shrugged his shoulders. "More's the pity." Raucous shouts from the tables caught his fleeting attentions. He turned to his companions. "Gentlemen, I believe the games await." He threw his arms around the men's shoulders and the three walked as one toward the tables. Wilmot looked back over his shoulder with a saucy glance. "More's the pity, indeed."

Pippa pulled Simon down to her height. "Serious men terrify the king. Foolish and amusing ones make him laugh," she whispered, dryly. "Those three cause him hysterics."

Simon watched them retreat, dumbfounded at the entire exchange. "Of that, I have no doubt."

"Lady Dillworth?" interrupted a shy courtesan.

Pippa turned to see a pretty, young girl standing before her. "Yes?"

"The countess desires another round, Milady."

Pippa turned to Simon with a rueful smile. "It appears I must leave you, Doctor. Would you care to join the men at the tables?"

"I am afraid I do not possess the requisite knowledge, Milady." He glanced toward an empty chair before the hearth and lifted his coupe. "Perhaps I shall finish my wine by the fire."

"As you like." She waved to a footman standing by the doorway. "More champagne, please."

At that, Pippa disappeared, leaving Simon alone in the crowd. Resigned, he took a seat by the fireplace and stared at the droplets that collected on the outside of his glass.

"May I join you?"

Simon looked up to see a smartly dressed, older gentleman standing before him. "Please." Simon gestured to the empty chair next to him.

"I confess I heard you introduced as Doctor McKensie."

Simon closed his eyes and groaned inwardly.

"No, no. I do not wish to trouble you with an affliction. I am Robert Boyle, alchymist to the King. Are you perhaps

McKensie, the physick who achieved such notable survival rates during the plague?"

Simon jumped to his feet. "Master Boyle, author of "The Skeptical Chymist"?"

"You are familiar?" Boyle asked, pleasantly surprised.

"I have read your book several times over, sir. I…I am indeed Simon McKensie, sir," stuttered Simon, astonished that the venerable scien'tist knew of him.

"You flatter me, Doctor. I am especially glad to have introduced myself. Your results made quite the sensation at Oxford."

Simon blushed. "Thank you, sir."

Boyle thought a moment. "Perhaps you would share your methods with us in person one day."

"I would like that very much indeed, sir," said Simon.

"I am in London, at Gresham Collage until the end of the month. Perhaps April or May?"

"I would be honored."

"In the meantime, I wonder if you are acquainted with the scientific chamber the king maintains in the basement. 'Tis something of an alchymist's laboratory. The king has a penchant for science and has been experimenting with mercury and its properties."

"I was unaware that the king holds an interest in scientific pursuits."

"He does, indeed. His interests lay firstly in alchemy and astronomy, and yet, he has a fascination with scientific investigation in all disciplines. I had hoped to speak with him about financing a patent, but it appears he will not be in attendance tonight." Boyle thought for a moment. "Since you seem to be as uninterested in gambling as I, perhaps you might enjoy a visit belowstairs?"

"You are very kind, sir. I would, indeed."

As they entered the ladies salon, Boyle set his arm to Simon's, stopping him short. They watched as a footman stole up to the games table. Tensed in anticipation of a rapid retreat, the footman seemed to know that the news he was about to impart would surely cause an excitable, if not volcanic reaction. Well used to her temper, the footman—and the guests—often departed much the worse for wear in these equations. Boyle seemed to know well, for he, too held his ground. The footman took a deep breath, then leaned down to the countess and whispered in her ear.

Pippa and the rest of the courtesans seated around the table looked away discreetly, gripping their cards in anticipation. They were not disappointed, for the countess let loose with a howl that set the footman back on his heels in defense of his hearing.

"Bastard!" The countess's cards flew into the air as the she slammed both hands upon the tabletop, rattling the coins at play. She stood, absorbing the full weight of the news. "I will have him to his knees in forgiveness!" At that, the Countess of Castlemaine gathered her costly skirts and stormed from the chamber. Several wary courtesans followed in her wake.

Simon looked to Boyle in alarm. "What has happened?"

Boyle turned to Simon with regret. "I'm afraid the evening is over before it has even begun."

CHAPTER THIRTY-ONE

"I WOULD RATHER DIE IN THE ADVENTURE
OF NOBLE ACHIEVEMENTS THAN LIVE IN
OBSCURE AND SLUGGISH SECURITY."
~ LADY MARGARET CAVENDISH

Bealeton House
St. James Parish, London
5 March 1667

Catherine sat quietly across the dining table from Simon in a soft pool of light from a single candelabrum, lost in thought. Simon was equally silent. He leaned back in the chair, his arms crossed, reflecting on the disastrous evening. Catherine gazed down the great length of the table in the dim, paneled dining hall, remembering the night of her engagement party to Miles when all twenty-four candelabras had been lit. Both the effect and the evening itself had been spectacular. Amidst the sparkling, high-spirited party, Aunt Viola had orchestrated a Bride's Pie triumph, astounding everyone with twenty-four live birds escaping wildly from the enormous baked vessel. Simon had been an unexpected guest at the dinner party. Uncomfortable and shy in such glittering, aristocratic company, he had stayed for just one dance before giving her a copy of his book and slipping into the night. Catherine had stayed awake all night reading, consumed by both his intellect and his medical research, and by the morning light, she knew in her heart that she would never marry Miles. That night seemed so very long ago.

Simon leaned forward on the table. "Is this what you wish for your life, Catherine?" he said, his voice weary and soft.

"To consort with these people? Because in truth, I confess to finding nearly every man I met this night, all but contemptible. I am nae political, nor do I wish to pass a moral judgment upon the king who's circle seems to be filled with an appalling excess of women, sport and debauchery, but neither do I wish to curry favor with such a man to advance my position. My God, Catherine, the whole of London lies in ashes and ruin, yet you would not know it from the senseless folly I witnessed this night."

Catherine leaned on an elbow and contemplated his displeasure with a sinking heart.

"Even Robert Boyle was a willing actor in the farce. As accomplished a man of science that he is, must he curry favor with the king to advance this knowledge? Is the king's purse that much of a prize that he would consort willingly with such dandies and fools?" mused Simon. He flexed his feet in his leather boots and stretched out once more in the dainty wooden chair. The chair cracked beneath him, startling them both. Simon jumped to his feet. "I am not meant for such fine furniture!" he cried in frustration, as he fell to his knees and examined the wood for damage.

Catherine blew softly on the candle, and watched the flame waver as she collected her thoughts. "I was disappointed in the evening, myself."

Simon stopped short, looking up to her with a mixture of surprise and relief. He exhaled, his anger quickly dissipating. "I…I apologize for my ill humor, Catherine. In all honesty, I was unsure as to whether you wished to belong in that world, rather than the one to which I belong." He moved to another chair.

Catherine ran her fingers over a scratch in the wood. "I ran from that world, Simon, the day I broke the engagement to Miles." She looked away, as though troubled by an embarrassing confession. "I only wished to become better acquainted with Elizabeth and the ladies in her circle, as they are all very accomplished women.

I have so enjoyed our weekly gatherings." She faced Simon with a sadness he had not before seen. "I thought perhaps I might learn from the woman they associate with as well, but tonight, I found that have I nothing to learn from those who surround the duchess at court. Those women are consumed with gossip. They can speak of nothing else but frivolous talk of hair or the latest dress designs from Paris."

MaryPryde entered with tea and sweets on a tray. "Beggin' your pardon. 'Tis from the kitchen, Milord. Gussie thought ye's might be a bit peckish," she said, setting the tray on the table.

Simon acknowledged MaryPryde with a grateful nod, and then turned back to Catherine. "I fear that with the exception of Mr. Boyle, the men were no better," he said, with all the restraint his good manners could muster.

Catherine stared into the candleflame. "I wish to do something useful with my life, Simon, the way Elizabeth and her friends have. They will all leave behind something of value for having been on this earth—something that has made another's life easier, or perhaps, more enjoyable."

Listening intently, MaryPryde poured the tea.

"Is architecture a discipline you wish to master? Perhaps we could arrange…?"

"No, Simon. I am grateful for your offer, but I have found that it is not. Although I have been fascinated by all I have learned and am grateful for knowledge, I find that I am far more interested in science and the natural world."

Simon looked confused. "If that is your interest, why have you not returned to the dissectory?"

She looked up from the candle and stared at him. "Do you not know?"

"I am afraid I…I do not," he said, furrowing his brow.

"Dr. Palgrave has made it more than clear that I am not welcome." Her voice began to shake in anger and humiliation. "As a woman, I am of no use to him or the hospital."

He reached across the table and took her hands in his. "Nothing could be farther from the truth," he said, his earnest eyes searching hers. "You and your talents are of very great use. Your being a woman has no bearing on your abilities, Catherine."

Catherine began to calm down. "There are many who would disagree."

Simon shook his head. "Dr. Palgrave is no longer in charge, and you would certainly be welcomed back by Father Hardwicke." He cocked his eyebrow and smiled. "Most especially if you offer aid in raising the stature of—and donations to—the hospital by illustrating the research we conduct in the dissectory."

At that, her good humor returned. "With Father Hardwicke championing my work, I might indeed return," she said, her gray eyes sparkling at the prospect.

Much relieved, Simon laughed. "Just please, please promise that there will be no more presentations at court for a very long time," he grinned, removing the court wig. "I am uncomfortable in the extreme at those ridiculous gatherings." He gave Catherine a rueful glance. "Perhaps, however, with the king championing my own work, I might already have found a volunteer for the experiment."

MaryPryde fingered the leaflet she carried in the pocket of her apron still. She looked to Simon as though to speak, then caught her tongue. She turned back to her tray of sweets.

"You have not yet found a willing soul?" asked Catherine.

"Nae, not a one," he shook his head, weary at the thought.

"Perhaps if you increased the offering? I can speak to the solicitor in the morning—Father made arrangements…"

"I am grateful for your offer, and yet I should think that three gold crowns would be more than enough to entice. Why, the city is full of men in need."

"Is it a *man* that you require?" blurted MaryPryde, holding back no longer. She ducked her head. "Pardon me, Milord," she whispered.

Simon was taken off guard. "I beg your pardon, what did you say?"

MaryPryde pulled the leaflet from her apron pocket and held it out. "Is it a man that you require, sir?" She pointed to the leaflet. "If not, might I offer myself?" MaryPryde lifted her chin in defiance. "I wish to do something important with me own life, just as Lady McKensie has."

Simon looked to Catherine, as if to contemplate the propriety of such a course. "I do not know whether..." He paused, and then tried again to express the thoughts roiling in his mind. "Is it proper that a woman be the subject of such an experiment?"

MaryPryde stood tall. "Did ye not say that a woman could be equal in ability? If you meant yer words, then I should be of equal value to you, sir."

"I did, indeed, MaryPryde. Yet, I do not believe that you understand what the experiment entails."

"I have heard ye speak of it, Milord. 'Tis a blood trans... trans..." She wrinkled her brow in thought. "I canna' remember th' name, but I do understand."

"It is a blood transfusion experiment, MaryPryde, and as it is an experiment, you must realize that there can be no guaranty of your safety."

She considered the prospect for a moment, and then steeled her shoulders. "I dinna' care."

"Are you certain, MaryPryde?" asked Catherine, concerned for them both.

"I am, Milady. I'm grateful to ye for the position here at Bealeton House," she paused a moment before speaking out, "but I wish to 'ave me own dressmaking stall at the Exchange, an' with three gold crowns, I can buy me own fabric and let the stall." She backed away, embarrassed by her confession.

"MaryPryde, we would be happy to help you in any way…."

"Nae, Miss. Thank ye, but I'll not be obliged to anyone, even for such a generous offer. Me father weren't kin t' charity. We earn our own, he'd say. A'course, if ye'd allow me to stay on while I set up shop, I'd be grateful to ye, Milady." She busied herself pouring more tea.

"We would be happy to have you stay on, MaryPryde. You will always have a home here."

MaryPryde looked as if she might cry. "Oh, thank ye miss," she whispered.

Catherine cradled the steaming cup with both hands and contemplated the candle flame's reflection in the tea. "You must do everything in this life you wish," she said, softly. Catherine glanced to MaryPryde and smiled. "Those were the last words my father spoke, MaryPryde. He said one must do everything in life they wished."

"It is me own wish," said MaryPryde, with a stubborn set to her chin.

Catherine reached across the table and set her hand upon Simon's. "Then, we have no right to stand in her path," she said.

Simon felt the weight of the world lift from his shoulders. "Very well, then. We shall check you in to the hospital tomorrow night, with the understanding that you may change your mind at any moment."

"I'll not change me mind, Milord," MaryPryde assured him. "I'll nae go back on me word." She took up the tray and left the dining room, smiling at the delicious thought of three gold crowns jangling in her pockets.

CHAPTER THIRTY-TWO

MaryPryde spent a quiet day before the experiment dutifully reciting her Sunday prayers in church, and then, as night fell, Simon and Catherine escorted her in the family carriage to the hospital. Happily wriggling her toes under a new set of crisp, clean linens, MaryPryde glanced to Sister Rosamond and stifled a giggle of excitement at the adventure that lay ahead. Simon had taken all possible measures for MaryPryde's comfort. The dissection table had been moved out, and a rope bed installed in its place. A feather mattress from the nun's quarters had been laid over the ropes, creating a soft, cozy nest to lie upon during the experiment that would last nearly two days. A simple chair for Sister Rosamond had been placed near the bed.

MaryPryde lay back on the pillow and sighed a contented sigh feeling very much like a fine lady of the manor. She lifted the ruffled sleeve of the gown and robe given to her by Catherine as a gift and examined the tight, even stitches and the way the heavy fabric laid soft upon her skin. She marveled at the gown's fine workmanship, hardly believing that she was in such extravagant nightclothes.

Sister Rosamond set MaryPryde's valise on a stool with a thud, and then moved the stool next to the bed. "Ye might be needing yer things," said Sister Rosamond. She moved a cloth-covered basket to the illustration table. Lifting a corner of the cloth, she peeked inside. It was filled with a loaf of bread, a jar of jam, and several cuts of dried beef. "'Tis a lovely tatter ye brought."

"Aye, Gussie sent it." MaryPryde smiled softly, thinking of the cook. As plain spoken as she was, Gussie had a very tender heart and had taken MaryPryde under her wing as though she were her very own. "She feared ye wouldna' feed me."

Sister Rosamond fussed with the basket. "There's no need to fret, Miss. As ye can tell, we intend t' take very good care of ye nae."

And, indeed, they had. For the last two hours, MaryPryde had been weighed, then measured by a team of nuns, each measurement carefully notated into a small ledger by Simon. She had then been treated to a hearty supper of roast chicken and pottage, as well as a small loaf of bread and tea. The feast was followed by a brisk wash down by Sister Rosamond. MaryPryde pulled the quilt closer to her chin and reveled in what felt in her limited imaginings something very much akin to a holiday.

Before leaving to assemble his instruments for the following morning's experiment, Simon delivered on his promise, and MaryPryde's bag now jangled with three brand-new gold crowns. As night fell, she laid her head on the down pillow and sighed a contented sigh. Never in her life had she been the focus of such fussing attentions.

"Are ye chilled, Miss?" asked Sister Rosamond, lighting the torches along the walls of the theater. "Would ye care fer another quilt?"

MaryPryde thought of the filthy snow melting outside the hospital and shivered. "Aye, Sister. I would."

Sister Rosamond smiled as she unfurled another quilt over the girl. "Another pillow, perhaps?"

"Aye, Sister, I would, indeed," grinned MaryPryde. "'Tis kind of ye to treat me so well."

Sister Rosamond placed another pillow behind MaryPryde's head. "Nonsense," she said briskly. "Dr. McKensie has given orders that ye be well taken care of during your stay here, and that is precisely what I intend to do." She leaned over the bed, smoothing the quilt. "Yer quite brave, you know," said Sister Rosamond, lifting an eyebrow.

MaryPryde turned away, humbled by the thought. "The doctor and Lady McKensie have been very good to me. I could see 'e were troubled, an' I…I wanted to help."

Sister Rosamond set the flint in her pocket, and then removed her Nuremberg spectacles. Squinting, she held them under the torchlight. "'Tis an awful thing to grow old and need these cursed things to see." She rubbed at a smudge on the glass with her tunic, and then held them up to the light once more. "Still an' all, they're a bit of a miracle, aren't they?" She idly rubbed at the glass again. "Yer a good girl, Miss." She looked closely at each lens, this time, satisfied. "Are ye at all afraid?

MaryPryde furrowed her brow. "I dinna' think so. Would ye be?"

Sister Rosamond put her spectacles back on, and then took hold of a small wooden cross she wore on a rope around her waist. "I have faith, MaryPryde," the nun smiled. "Therefore do not worry about tomorrow, for tomorrow will worry about itself," she smiled. "Matthew 6:34." Sister Rosamond tucked the quilts around MaryPryde, and then settled herself into the chair by the bed. She reached for her bible. "Nae get some sleep, Miss, for tomorrow will be here soon enough, indeed."

❦

Monday, 7 March 1667
8:30am

Quiet murmurings of a new day drifted into the dissectory, as the hospital slowly came to life. Orderlies threaded their way between the rows of rope pallets handing out bowls of porridge to the sleepy patients in the great hall. In the soft dissectory bed, MaryPryde was enjoying the last of her own breakfast porridge as Catherine and Simon came into the room. She set the spoon down and moved the tray aside. "Good morning, Milady, Milord," she smiled.

"How are you this morning, MaryPryde?" asked Catherine, handing the empty breakfast tray to a waiting orderly.

"Did you sleep well?" asked Simon, looking through the ledger notes he had made the day before.

MaryPryde watched the orderly leave. She looked for Sister Rosamond, but her chair was empty. They were alone in the theater. Simon sat down on the edge of the bed, his eyes soft with concern.

"I did, Milord."

Simon made a brief notation of her slumber in the ledger, and then turned to give MaryPryde his full attention. "Lady McKensie and I wished to speak with you privately, before Father Hardwicke and the students arrive to observe the experiment. I would like to explain the procedure a bit more fully, but before I do, it is important for you to know that you are in no way bound to continue if you have even the slightest of misgivings. This is a scientific experiment, not a necessity, and you may stop the experiment at any time you wish, even after we have begun. Do you understand?"

"I do, Milord."

"Very well, then, we will proceed with the experiment as planned. When we begin, I will let blood from your right arm. I will not withdraw as much as is customarily drawn when there is an illness, however, as this is only an experiment. After a short interval, I will replace an equal amount of blood back into your left arm. That blood will come from a sheep."

MaryPryde's eyes widened, but she said nothing.

"The reason I am attempting this experiment is because I have a theory, an idea, if you will, that in some cases death results because far too much blood has been lost. If it is possible to replace that lost blood with no harm to the patient, lives may be saved. You are here to prove, or disprove, the theory that blood may be transfused from one living creature to another with no harm caused.

"Does that make sense, MaryPryde?" asked Catherine.

"Aye, it does."

Catherine hesitated. "And, if it is a question of the three crowns, you must know that arrangements can be made to establish you at the Exchange," she said. "We would be more than happy to help you."

"I'll not take charity, Milady. I intend to earn me own way."

A flash of relief crossed Simon's face. "Then, do you wish to continue?" he asked, his voice gentle.

MaryPryde thought of the dressmaking stall, of the bundles of fabrics she could buy, of the new life she would start with the payment. "I do, Milord," she said, with absolute certainty.

Simon stood. "Very well, MaryPryde. Rest a while longer. I will bring the medical students in soon."

∽∾

12:00pm

Simon removed a clean cloth from a tray of instruments next to the bedstead. As the acrid scent of the vinegar that covered the instruments wafted through the small chamber, his thoughts were instantly overwhelmed by memories of Wells. *Could he have saved more of them?* The thoughts haunted him still. Simon breathed deeply to clear his mind. Focusing on the task ahead, he set both hands deep into the vinegar for a moment. Simon took hold of a second cloth and dipped it in the liquid, then wiped MaryPryde's outstretched arm with it. MaryPryde wrinkled her nose and turned her head from the sharp smell. Handing the cloth to Sister Rosamond, Simon reached into the tray once more and took hold of his tortoise shell lancet. As he wiped it dry, he wondered if the students assembled on the viewing platform could see his hands shaking.

"Why the vinegar, Doctor?" called out one of the students. "Good Lord, it reeks to the heavens."

Father Hardwicke stepped in, speaking pointedly to the inquiring student. "If you have given Doctor McKensie's research any attention at all, Master Jenkins, you will no doubt have learned that his views on medical practices are quite different than other physicks on staff."

Simon looked at the fifteen students on the viewing platform staring at him expectantly and stopped a moment to elaborate. "Though I cannot say why, I believe that cleanliness contributes to healing. Current research from the University of Leiden confirms that same belief. Through careful and recorded observations during both the plague in Wells and here in the hospital, I have seen time and again that the filthy practices of others can cause further injury and infection. Therefore, in both my research and in my daily practice, I believe in the use of vinegar as a disinfecting quality for both the flesh, and the instruments I use." He nodded to the attentive medical students. "We shall proceed."

Concentrating on MaryPryde once again, Simon glanced first to Catherine at her table illustrating each step of the experiment, and then to Father Hardwicke, who stood across the bed watching his every move with a mixture of pride and curiosity.

Father Hardwicke gave an encouraging nod. "Carry on."

"Are you ready, Miss Beckwith?" Simon asked, the scalpel point pressing into the soft flesh of her forearm. "This will hurt a moment."

MaryPryde drew a big breath. "Aye, I am, Milord. Go on, then."

Simon glanced at a small glass vessel positioned on the floor beneath MaryPryde's hand, and then withdrew the lancet. He glanced to the students.

"Haggett!"

Crushed in the center of the viewing stand, every muscle in Oswold's body seized in reflexive fear. *What had he done now?* Heads jerked toward him from all directions, focusing an unusual amount of curiosity on the fumbling medical student. He broke into a sweat. "Aye, sir," he stammered, wary of the sudden attention from his peers.

"I believe I would prefer a student hold the vessel while I perform the venesection. Will you assist?"

"Aye, sir!" breathed Oswold, his eyes wide, incredulous at being favorably singled out. He gazed at the students around him. A sudden swagger made him stand tall for the moment. He took a step. The astonished students on the viewing stand moved aside to allow him a path to the bedstead. Slightly off balance, Oswold caught the heel of his boot descending the platform, and collided with Father Hardwicke. Jenkins and a few of the other students laughed into the sleeves of their tunics.

"Beg your pardon, Father," Oswold mumbled as he stepped back, his cheeks a virulent shade of crimson. The swagger was gone.

Father Hardwicke set the young man to rights with a slight smile. "Over there, Haggett," he said, pointing toward a tray of lancets and linen strips.

"Aye," Oswold said, much humbled. He took his place next to Simon.

Simon picked up the glass and held it out toward to the students. "As you can see, I have etched several markings into the glass." He pointed to a series of measured, inscribed lines. "We will collect just enough to reach the second mark." Simon turned back to Oswold. "Hold this glass at her wrist and collect the blood into the vessel. Call out when the second marker has been reached."

"Aye, sir." As Oswold took hold of the glass, it slipped in his sweaty palm. He quickly secured the vessel with his other hand to the groans of the students who were suddenly quite jealous of his good fortune.

Coming to his defense, Father Hardwicke raised an eyebrow, silencing the criticisms. "Enough."

Nestled deep under the pile of quilts, MaryPryde looked up to Oswold and smiled, her eyes crinkling at the corners. Turning bright crimson, Oswold ducked his head, enchanted by both her smile and her golden-green eyes. *No maid had ever smiled at him.* He took a deep breath, gathered his wits and readied the vessel.

Simon held the lancet just above the skin of MaryPryde's right forearm. He could see the dull, dark blue veins tracing just below the pale, translucent surface. Choosing the thickest of the veins, Simon set the razor sharp point to the flesh and, glancing to MaryPryde to assure himself once more of her willingness, pressed down. The lancet slid smoothly through the skin.

MaryPryde took a sharp breath. She gripped the quilts with her left hand and groaned, but did not cry out. Sister Rosamond dipped a cloth in a bowl of cool water and laid it across MaryPryde's forehead.

"Yer a courageous lass," Sister Rosamond said, her voice soft and soothing. She nodded toward the viewing platform. "These gentlemen would sink to their knees, like as not," she whispered. MaryPryde stifled a giggle.

The small incision made, Simon lifted the blade and set the lancet into the tray of vinegar, then looked back to MaryPryde's arm. Dark red blood billowed to the surface, filling the cut until it at last overflowed. The students were mesmerized. A deep line of crimson began to trickle down her forearm inch by inch until it reached the wrist. There, the languid line began to slowly encircle the wrist bone. The blood collected underneath into a tremulous, glossy globule until it could hold together no more. Then, one drop fell. *Drip.* Oswold's hands shook as the blood began to stain the bottom of the glass. *Drip.* More blood began to fall from her wrist. *Drip.* The students watched intently as the thick liquid collected in the vessel. It began to rise steadily toward the first marker. *Drip.*

Catherine, having completed a sketch of the entire scene, began to illustrate a closer view of the venesection. She rose to take a measurement of the narrow incision, and then went back to her drawing table. The arm's length and circumference measurements had been taken the night before, and while the main sketches would be drawn in the dissectory, Catherine would add in the finer details after the experiment ended. The silence in the room was palpable as the students watched the blood level rise in the glass. They had all seen bloodlettings many times before, but the theater of this particular experiment, the girl, the sheep, the transfusion, had them spellbound. Even Father Hardwicke could not take his eyes from the blood collecting in the glass.

"Marker one!" cried Oswold.

The students took a collective breath and inched forward on the platform, straining to watch the level rise.

"Blasphemous!"

Heads jerked toward the doorway. There, Dr. Godfrey Palgrave stood, shaking in outrage. "'Tis a damnable sin, what you do here this day!" he cried.

MaryPryde looked to Simon in alarm, instinctively terrified by the unsettling sight of the unkempt man shouting from the doorway. His tunics were covered in blood, his hair hung long and stringy. He stood in stark contrast to Simon and the students around her. She fought the urge to scream.

Father Hardwicke stepped in. "Palgrave? What business have you here?"

Palgrave grabbed the arm of a young man and pulled him into the doorway. "The boy says he has a delivery for McKensie."

The delivery boy wrenched his arm from Palgrave's grasp. He held a basket in his other arm. "Morley and Son's Butcher's Shop, sir. "Mr. Morley said I 'ad to deliver by one o'clock sharp."

"A butcher shop?" shouted Palgrave. "What possible trade do you conduct here?!"

Father Hardwicke calmly checked his pocket watch, then walked over to the delivery boy and took the basket in hand. "And 'tis indeed precisely one o'clock." He clapped the boy on his shoulder. "Well done, lad. See the registrar on your way out. Tell him I said to give you two shillings for your trouble."

"Two? Aye, I will!" The boy grinned, nodded his gratitude and ran from the dissectory, hat in hand.

Palgrave looked as though he would mount yet another condemnation. Father Hardwicke stopped him. "No more."

Spurned once again, Palgrave balled his trembling fists, and then pounded one into the other in contemplation of the entire unholy enterprise. "May the Lord God curse you all!" In sheer animus, Godfrey leaned into the room and spit on the floor before walking on.

Disgusted, Simon looked to an orderly standing nearby. "Get a cloth and clean that up, please." Simon glanced to a wide-eyed MaryPryde. "How do you feel? Do you wish to continue?"

"I do," she said quietly, though clearly unsettled by the unexpected outburst.

"He'll not return," reassured Simon. "I shall see to it."

Through it all, Oswold had not taken his eyes from the vessel for one moment. "Second marker!" he cried out.

An excited murmur of anticipation rippled through the students. Simon reached for the strips of linen and bound the wound tightly, then looked to MaryPryde. "Half done. Let's take a moment, shall we?" She gave him a grateful smile. He turned to Sister Rosamond standing at the bedside. "Perhaps a sip of water for Miss Beckwith?"

"Aye, Dr. McKensie! A sip of water, indeed," said Sister Rosamond, a bit addled by all she had seen. She quickly turned from the bed to fuss with the bucket and ladle, for she too, had been transfixed.

As Sister Rosamond gave MaryPryde the water, Simon took the delivery basket in hand. From it, he removed a length of fresh sheep gut, a sheep's bladder and a vessel of fresh sheep's blood and laid it all on the table next to the tray. As he had practiced, Simon made a deft incision in the bladder and set it aside. He took a length of twine and bound one end of the intestine to the wide end of the fattest goose quill, then took a scalpel and cut the gut to a cubit—the length from his fingertip to his elbow. He stretched the opposite end around the sheep's bladder. Once the bladder was secure, he made a wide incision at the top. Father Hardwicke and the students stared in open-mouthed wonder at the sight that was unfolding

Jenkins once again stepped to the edge of the platform. "One more question, sir," he dared. "Why use a sheep? Why not allow one of us to let our own blood?"

Simon looked up and paused, bladder in hand. "This is but the first in, I hope, a series of experiments of blood exsanguination and subsequent transfusion. I have studied the notes and procedures of Sir Richard Lower of Oxford for months in order to conduct this experiment, and while Sir Richard experiment was performed *canis autem canis*, dog to dog, as it were, that experiment has been successful. This is the first transfusion experiment involving a human being. *Animus autem hominum.* Animal to human. A butchered sheep was merely more convenient than a live dog," he explained. "Should this experiment also have a successful outcome, the next attempt will be *hominun autem hominem.*

For the first time, MaryPryde looked unsettled. "My apologies, Miss Beckwith. There is no reason to expect anything but a successful outcome today," reassured Simon. He glanced to Father Hardwicke, a fleeting expression of irritation crossing his brow.

"Are there any further questions?" asked Father Hardwicke, anxious to keep MaryPryde as calm as possible. "If not, perhaps we might proceed?" Jenkins slunk back into the crowd. He had no more questions.

Simon produced a second glass vessel with etched markings. He turned to Oswold, and gestured to the vessel of blood from the butcher. "Perhaps you would measure the blood to the second mark?" The medical students to a man took a collective breath in anticipation of an impending disaster. Oswold himself, looked terribly unsure. Simon nodded his encouragement.

"As you wish, Doctor McKensie." Simon watched as the trembling Oswold poured the sheep's blood into the empty vessel. He stopped at exactly the second mark.

"Well done, Haggett."

As the students exhaled, Simon poured the contents of the etched vessel inside the sheep's bladder and again, secured the opening with twine. Blood ran down through the sheep's gut and spilled from the quill before Simon blocked the opening with his finger. He held the entire apparatus up for all to see. The students crowded the platform, straining to get a better view.

"May I take measurements?" asked Catherine.

"Haggett, place your hands in the vinegar, and then hold the device for Lady McKensie while I prepare for the incision in Miss Beckwith's left arm."

Oswold dipped his hands in the vinegar and then carefully placed his finger over the quill opening as he took the device to the illustration table. Catherine took a length of marked twine and measured the quill, the length of sheep's gut, and the girth of the bladder. She made notes on the parchment for the drawing that would come next, then nodded to Simon.

Simon set his hands into the tray once more, and then wiped a vinegar soaked cloth across MaryPryde's arm. He took the lancet back in hand and gave her a smile. "Shall we proceed?"

"Aye, Milord," came the determined reply.

Simon found the thick blue vein and pressed the lancet in. MaryPryde squeezed her eyes shut, gritting her teeth as he pulled it back out. The blood saturated the wound, but this time, Simon pressed a cloth down on the incision. "Haggett!"

Oswold stepped to the bedstead with the apparatus. He handed Simon the quill, spilling a drop in the transfer. The students leaned in to watch as Simon removed the cloth. A bit of blood spilled once more as Simon inserted the quill into the incision, though it was unclear as to whose blood it was, MaryPryde's or the sheep's. MaryPryde winced as the quill went in, but she too, was fascinated. Simon took the bladder from Oswold and held it high.

"How much are ye putting in, if I might ask, Milord?" whispered MaryPryde.

"The marks on the glass are equal to two spoonfuls of liquid. I do not expect that all will be absorbed, however."

The room fell silent once more as the blood dripped with the force of gravity into MaryPryde's arm. The only sound in the silent chamber was the scratching of Catherine's illustration quill on parchment. MaryPryde stared at her arm, watching as blood spilled from the wound. "D'yes think much of it's going inside?"

"Aye, I do. Enough for our purposes today."

After what seemed an eternity, the blood stopped flowing through the sheep gut. Simon removed the quill and bound the wound. He put the rigged device back into the basket and held it toward Oswold. "Haggett, dispose of this, if you would."

"Aye, Doctor," he said, taking the basket in hand.

"And, Haggett?"

Oswold turned back, wary. "Aye, sir?"

"Well done."

Oswold swelled with pride.

Simon thought a moment. "Sister Rosamond will sit with MaryPryde until nine o'clock, after which time, I will stay the watch through the night. Until then, I intend to return to the administration office to document the procedure while it is top of mind. Haggett, might I ask you to remain with Sister Rosamond?"

Oswold dared a glance to MaryPryde. A broad grin spread across his face. "I would be most happy to, sir!" He grabbed hold of the basket, and walked from the dissectory with jounce to his step and a cheeky nod to the remaining students on the platform.

Simon faced the viewing stand. "And with endless gratitude to Miss Beckwith, that, gentlemen, is that. Please return to your duties."

CHAPTER THIRTY-THREE

"REVENGE, AT FIRST SWEET, BITTER ERE
LONG, BACK ON ITSELF RECOILS."
~ JOHN MILTON

St. Bartholomew's Hospital
Smithfield Parish, London
Monday, 7 March 1667
4:07pm

Catherine collected her drawing instruments, carefully storing her quills into a small wooden box at the side of the illustration table. It had been a long day, and although she was bone-weary, she was well satisfied that she had captured every step of the experiment on the parchments. The fine details were to be filled in later. Suddenly struck by an odd warmth that made her strangely lightheaded for a moment, Catherine reached over and filled a cup from the water bucket. She took a cooling sip. T'was a very long day, indeed. She looked at MaryPryde lying quietly in the bed watching her and smiled. "Would you like to see the drawings?" she asked.

"Aye, I would, Milady."

Catherine brought the nine sketches she had made to the bedstead, showing first the large sketch of everyone in the room. She then held out the drawing of MaryPryde, herself. The rest of the illustrations, the close-up views of the device, the incisions and the procedure itself as it unfolded, were left on the table.

MaryPryde stared with interest at her portrait, as though she did not quite believe that she was the pretty girl in the picture. "'Tis a very favorable likeness, Milady."

"You're very pretty, MaryPryde."

MaryPryde stared a moment longer, then set the drawing aside and sighed. "I could never do what ye do."

"But, you see, you have other talents," smiled Catherine. "I could not design and sew a dress if I tried. I haven't the patience. I never have had it."

"I don't mean just yer drawings, Lady McKensie. Ye've done so much—ye've written a real book, the work with Lady Wilbraham, why, even what ye do here at the hospital. 'Tis a right wonder, t' be sure."

"You are very young, MaryPryde. I promise you will have plenty of time to do the things you wish to do, and I believe that you possess the will to do just that. Why, look at what you've done here today."

MaryPryde looked up at her with interest. "Beggin' your pardon, Milady?"

"You may think you simply volunteered to help Dr. McKensie, but you have in truth accomplished so much more, MaryPryde. You have made a contribution to medical science —a contribution that may well save many lives. Very few in this world can say that."

"A contribution to medical science that saves lives?" MaryPryde was shocked.

"Aye. Your name, should you wish it recorded, will be forever remembered."

"It will?" she whispered. MaryPryde gazed down in wonder at the coarse, linen dressings wound around both arms. "I would like that, Milady. I would like that very much," she said, her voice soft with emotion. She tucked a stray piece of linen back into the dressing as she absorbed the enormity of the thought, then looked up to Catherine. "T'was the fire, you know." She paused a moment. "It changed me life. I wouldn'a known you, ye see. The plague changed it first, a' course, but I would'na had the courage to chart me own course the way you do if the fire had'na happened. I wouldn'a known such a thing was even possible. I surely would'na be layin' here."

"I think the fire changed all our lives," said Catherine. "Some for the better, some for the worse, but there is no doubt that some good came from it."

MaryPryde pulled the quilts to her chin and giggled. "My name, forever remembered. Can ye imagine, Milady?"

"You should be very proud of yourself, MaryPryde. You have accomplished much for science. You have already made a difference in this world."

Tears filled MaryPryde's eyes. "I've made a difference," she whispered to herself, incredulous. "Thank you, Milady."

Catherine smiled, and then set the latch on her box of drawing instruments with a snap. "And now, I think you should get some rest. Doctor McKensie will be in soon to check on you."

"Yer leavin'?"

"I am, but I'll be here with Doctor McKensie. If you like, I will sit with you through the night."

"I would like that very much, Milady."

Sister Rosamond bustled into the room with a tea tray. She set it on the table by the bedstead, and then set her hand to MaryPryde's forehead. "No fevers. Good girl." She made a notation in the ledger, then straightened the bedclothes, and put the plate of biscuits on MaryPryde's lap. "Ye've got t' keep yer strength up," she said, pouring the tea.

Catherine put a gentle hand on MaryPryde's shoulder. "Get some rest, MaryPryde. The doctor and I will be back soon," she said, before leaving the chamber.

Crossing paths with Catherine, Oswold walked in carrying the ledger. He pulled a chair up to the bedstead, setting a quill and inkpot on the floor by the chair. He opened the ledger to the last entry and looked up expectantly. "I'm to sit with you, Sister."

Sister Rosamond turned away and silently crossed herself. "Lord, give me strength," she whispered. Turning back to face Oswold, she smiled brightly. "That will be lovely. Lovely, indeed."

8:38pm

I am getting old. Sister Rosamond sighed as she waited for Simon to return and take the watch. Her head ached beyond reckoning and she longed for her bed in the private quarters above the administration offices. She had spent hours listening to Oswold marvel over the experiment they that day witnessed. His endless deliberations on the method and outcome had finally worn her out. For some measure of relief, she had sent Oswold in search of evening collop for them both, and was grateful for the blessed silence in his absence. As promised, Simon had come back on the hour to record in his ledger any observed changes. She looked to MaryPryde sleeping soundly. *Thankfully, there had been no changes.*

In the quiet theater, Sister Rosamond extinguished all but one torch above her chair. Sitting under its soft glow, she reached for her bible as she reflected upon the day's extraordinary events. Despite the vociferous protestations of Dr. Palgrave, she had become well accustomed to the autopsies Simon performed, and yet this was something entirely different. She herself had no qualms about the dissections, knowing that her own medical knowledge had increased since Simon had been given authority to proceed, yet she knew there were others besides Palgrave who were violently opposed to the research on religious grounds. Nearly each to a man kept his own counsel, however, knowing the admiration Dr. Hardwicke had for the intelligent, young physick. At times, their opposition struck an arrow straight into the heart of her own religious convictions. She wondered if she were right in her ceaseless support of the lad's ideas.

She sighed and glanced to MaryPryde, still asleep in the bedstead. Proverbs, she thought. *Proverbs always gave solace to the conflict in her soul.* She leafed through the pages to 3:18, a favorite. *The heart of the discerning acquires knowledge, for the ears of the wise seek it out.* She leaned her head back in the chair and closed her eyes a moment. *She could always depend on Proverbs for wisdom.*

Oswold returned to the dissectory, carrying with him a small loaf of bread, a knife and a cup of tea on a tray. "'Tis all the kitchen would spare, Sister Rosamond." He set the tray on her lap.

The nun sat up, casting a wary glance toward MaryPryde who stirred in the bed, but did not awaken. Sister Rosamond set a finger to her lips in caution. "Oh, I should love a slice of bread and a bit of tea, true as I live, Oswold," she whispered. Sister Rosamond rose and took the knife in hand to cut the bread. "Aye!" she breathed, drawing the blade through both the crusty loaf and her left thumb. Blood began to drip from the wound, leaving large splatters on the floorboards.

Oswold jumped to move the tray and examine the cut, and then quickly ran around the bed to grab the spare strips of linen piled on the bedside table. Sister Rosamond held her thumb up to the torchlight, squinting through her spectacles to see the extent of the injury. "'Tis blurred," she whispered in frustration. She removed her glasses and tried to wipe the glass. Blood smeared across the lenses.

"Let me help you, Sister," said Oswold. He reached for her spectacles to wipe the blood and in his clumsy haste, dropped them to the floor. "Beggin' your pardon," he breathed. As he stepped back to retrieve them, Oswold froze at the sound of glass grinding beneath his feet. He bent down and then looked to the nun in red-faced horror, holding the twisted, empty frames in hand. "I...I apologize, Sister," he mumbled softly, bowing his head in misery.

Sister Rosamond wound one of the linen strips tightly around her thumb, and then set the rest on the floor by the chair. She sought to calm the lad. "'Tis nothing to worry over, Oswold. I have a spare pair upstairs in my quarters."

Oswold looked up with the hope of redemption. "Shall I retrieve them for you?"

"Nae!" she whispered, raising both palms in fear of the next calamity. "Nae," she reassured. "I'll just run upstairs. Won't be a tick," she said softly, as she gathered her skirts. Sister Rosamond glanced to MaryPryde. "She'll sleep, like as not—if you're quiet," she said, cocking an eyebrow as she left.

"Aye, Sister," he said, much chagrined. He took a seat in the chair and watched MaryPryde, still sleeping in the bedstead. *Aye, she was beautiful.* After several minutes, he exhaled, then laid his head back and closed his eyes to rest. A dark, threatening shadow fell across his face. Oswold opened his eyes to the broad back of Dr. Palgrave leaning over the bedstead.

"Wicked!" Palgrave cried, pointing an accusing finger at MaryPryde.

"Wicked and sinful ye are!"

MaryPryde jolted awake to the snarling, twisted face of Palgrave shouting just inches from her face. Disoriented, she screamed in terror and slid beneath the quilts to evade his deafening condemnations.

Oswold jumped from the chair and tore at Palgrave, trying to pull him away from the bedstead. The burly Palgrave threw him off, sending Oswold crashing into the wall. His shoulder knocked the iron torch from its hook. As it fell to the floor, the flames caught the spare linen strips by the chair, igniting the pile. In a moment of pure instinct, Oswold grabbed the bucket and threw the water onto the fire, then swung the bucket at Palgrave, hitting him in the head. He tried to pull Palgrave off once more, striking him repeatedly. "No!" Oswold cried. "Leave her be!"

Palgrave never felt the blows. He pulled the quilts from the bed. "'Tis a godless abomination what ye've done here today!" he shouted in full voice. "A godless abomination!" Palgrave jabbed an arthritic finger toward a terrified MaryPryde as he stood over the bedstead, condemning her to the infernal pits of Abaddon. "Then shall he say also unto them on the left hand, depart from me, ye cursed, into everlasting fire, prepared for the devil and his angels!" he thundered. MaryPryde screamed once more, then fell into a direful silence. Palgrave's voice trailed off as he began to back away from the bed in a slow, fearful retreat of a terrifying sight he had never before laid witness to.

Oswold looked from the demented Palgrave to MaryPryde. His eyes widened in fear, for the girl seemed to have been overtaken by a terrifying and unnatural force.

"'Tis the devil!" whispered Palgrave, pointing to the bed. MaryPryde began to shake from her head to her feet. Arching backwards on the linens, every muscle in her body jerked wildly as though she were being thrown about by an unseen hand. Her eyes rolled back in her head, the white orbs looking for all the world like a demon possessed. "'Tis the *devil*, I say!" roared Palgrave, collecting his wits. "Them yella' eyes are the very eyes of the devil, himself!" He cast his eyes about the room, desperately looking for something, anything to restrain the girl. Palgrave grabbed the pillow from beneath her head and thrust it across her face. "I'll not bear the sight of it!" he cried in abject terror.

"No!" cried Oswold. "Dr. Palgrave, NO!"

Jerking and bucking beneath his weight, MaryPryde's violent spasms nearly threw the burly Palgrave to the floor. He shoved down harder on the pillow. "Submit yourselves therefore to God! Resist the devil, and he will flee from ye!" he shouted.

MaryPryde tried to scream out, but the pillow muffled her cries. Palgrave bore down with all his might. "And, the great dragon was cast out! Satan, which deceiveth the whole world was cast out into the earth! Be gone, Satan!" he thundered, bereft of all reason.

Oswold tore at the thick arms holding the pillow in place. Too slight to pull Palgrave off, Oswold cried out in desperation.

"NO! Let her up, Doctor! Let her up!" he shouted.

Her screams grew weaker. Palgrave himself became possessed as he threw his full weight atop the seizing girl. Her spasms began to slow.

Oswold threw his arms around Palgrave, tearing at his clothes, trying to pull him away. "Get off of her!"

Palgrave threw Oswold to the floor with a deluded screech. "Leave me be! 'Tis Satan himself, and no mistake!" He pushed harder on the pillow.

Oswold looked to the pallet, tears streaming down his face. He scrambled to his feet and pulled at Palgrave's arms. "Let her breathe, Doctor. I beg of you," he cried. "Let her breathe."

Suddenly, a strange, almost sacred calm seemed to befall Palgrave. He bowed his head in quiet prayer, mumbling under his breath. "Amen," he whispered. At length, he let the pillow slide to the floor. In the flickering torchlight, the deathly silence was unbearable.

The quiet was broken by Oswold's gut-wracking sobs. He leaned on the wall and clutched at his stomach. "Aye, what have ye done, sir? By God's oath, what have ye done!" Oswold cried, gasping for air.

Palgrave snapped back to reality. He faced Oswold, outraged. "I have done nothing, Haggett! Nothing! 'Tis McKensie who's responsible for this girl's death!"

"Nae! 'Tis you who held the pillow down! Ye've killed her!"

Palgrave backslapped Oswold hard across the face. "Ye'll nae speak them words a'gin lest I curse ye to one side of hell and out th' other." He drew himself up to his full height. "I'll have ye cast from this place!" he screamed.

Oswold sagged against the wall, rubbing his palm across his aching jaw in sorrowful contemplation of a very bleak future. *His father would be ruined if he were to be expelled from medical school.* "What...what should I do?" he whispered.

Palgrave stepped past the wounded intern out to the hallway

that led into the great hall. "Guards!" he bellowed. "Summon the guards!" He turned to Oswold still in the dissectory, setting both hands on the plaster by the intern's ears. Palgrave leaned in. Oswold turned from his foul breath. "Speak not to a soul of this," he hissed, his voice low and threatening.

The hospital guards appeared at the doorway. "Aye?" they grunted, staring at the body of MaryPryde.

Palgrave went out to the hall and gestured wildly. "The administration offices! Arrest Simon McKensie...*on the charge of murder!*"

The guards turned as one and ran for the administration chambers. Palgrave returned to the dissectory. In the pale light leaking from the hallway, Palgrave took one last look at MaryPryde lying dead on the rope pallet. "Haggett!" he hissed. "Remove her." There was no response. "Haggett!" he cried out once more. He lit a torch and looked around the chamber. Godfrey Palgrave was alone.

CHAPTER THIRTY-FOUR

Tuesday, 8 March 1667
4:07am

With only the stars above to light his way, a terrified Oswold Haggett ran. With every desperate step, every heart-pounding breath, he left the hospital farther and farther behind. Midnight came and went, and still he ran. His feet ached. His head hurt. His lungs were about to burst as he tripped and scudded through the melting snows of the forests and fields toward Stockton Heath, a small village nearly twenty miles north of London. And still, hour after wretched hour, he ran.

No matter how hard he tried, Oswold could not banish from his mind the sight of MaryPryde lying dead. No matter how fast he ran he could not escape the gruesome deed. *He had laid witness to murder.* No matter how far or how long he ran, she was *there*. She had smiled at him. *No maid had ever smiled at him.* Tears flowing, he churned northward.

As the desolate night slipped toward a pale dawn, Oswold came upon a familiar brook. *He was not far from home.* The swiftly moving water splashed and tumbled against the rocks that lined the grassy banks. On the sloping berm, tiny woodland wildflowers were just beginning to bloom in the warmth of an early spring. The icy waters tempted. If he could just cool his feet a moment, he would have the strength to run the rest of the way home. *He would be safe at the farm.*

The sky had lightened to a dull cream when Oswold finally stopped running. Exhausted, he dropped to a moss-covered rock to catch his breath. After a moment, he unbuckled his boots and dipped his pale, blistered toes into a deep pool away from the tumbling stream. Staring into the clear, cold water, he could see the pebbles that had collected at the bottom. A falling twig landed on the still water with a delicate splash. As he watched it drift lazily downstream, the silence overwhelmed him. His anguished thoughts became desperate. *I could simply slip in and end this torment.* He leaned down and traced his finger through the water, leaving a tiny wake. *It would take but a moment. One single moment.* He suddenly thought of his father. He closed his eyes and sighed. *He could not do it.* Oswold sat up. Pulling his feet from the brook before they went numb, he shoved them them back into his boots, then splashed his face to clear his thoughts. He cupped his hands and, guzzling every drop, felt the icy water spill down his chin. She smiled at him. *No maid had ever smiled at him.* Reluctantly, Oswold stood. He wiped his jaw with the back of his hand and ran on.

The small, stone cottage was quiet. Soft, pink buds forming on the apple trees that fronted the cottage wavered in the early morning breeze. Even the chickens were asleep in their coop. He stared at the bright blue front door. Oswold thought of waking his father, but instead, he turned away. Picking a handful of spring grass, Oswold headed out to the barn. An old plow horse whinnied softly in the pasture as he closed the gate behind him, its gentle neigh at once so familiar, so comforting. He held the grass up and stroked it's long nose, savoring the soft nuzzles and quiet grunts as the horse chewed the verdant treat.

"Aye, Penderal," he whispered to the sturdy black gelding, "'tis a blessing to be a horse, is it not?"

Reluctantly leaving the horse behind, Oswold stole into the barn. Latching the door behind him, he climbed the ladder to the hayloft that was as wide as the barn itself. He slipped behind a mound of hay taller than he, and spread the straw flat, then laid down to rest as the morning sun at last broke through the very long night. *He was so tired.* As he drifted to sleep, the thick, sweet scent of hay that permeated the barn made his eyes tear up and spill over. *At least he thought it was the straw.*

CHAPTER THIRTY-FIVE

"EXCEPT BY THE LAWFUL JUDGMENT OF HIS
PEERS OR BY THE LAW OF THE LAND"
~ MAGNA CARTA 1215 AD

The Public Office
Bow Street Magistrate
London, England
Tuesday, 8 March 1667
2:52 pm

Simon shuffled before the magistrate of the Public
Office, the judge who would rule as to whether he
would be released or bound over for trial, to the raucous cries
from the crowd of onlookers. His ankles and feet were bloodied
from the tightly bound shackles. His tunics were filthy, as was
he from his long night on the floor in Caroome House where
prisoners were taken after the fire destroyed both Newgate and
Old Bailey prisons. Not once in his life had he felt so helpless
or humiliated. He dared a glance to Catherine standing in the
back of the room. He had brought such disgrace to her. She
looked tired and pale in the crowded, airless room. He knew
she had not slept the night before, not since the guards burst
into the administration office and seized him, pulling him
through the streets in chains.

"Silence!" cried the judge. He sat at a wide, wooden table
looking over the hastily written indictment. Off to the side, at a
small table, a gaunt, bespectacled man sat, quill in hand, poised
to transcribe the proceedings. After a long moment, the august
magistrate gazed around the room to the witnesses and onlookers.
"We assemble in Sessions this day to hear the charges against this

defendant and to determine if the evidence offered is sufficient to bind the defendant over for trial." He leveled his gaze to the onlookers. "Who here stands in accusation of this man?"

"I do, Milord," came a shout from the back of the room.

"Name?"

Palgrave shoved his way through the spectators to the front of the crowd. "Dr. Godfrey Palgrave."

The bespectacled man scribbled on the parchments.

"On what charge say you?" commanded the magistrate.

Palgrave paused a moment, waiting for all eyes to turn his way. He raised his voice as loud as he could. "I charge the physick, Simon McKensie, with both the murder of the young woman, MaryPryde Beckwith…" He turned to face Simon, who stood alone, his head lowered in shame, "…and the felonious crimes of grave-robbing, exhumation and the illegal dissection and dismemberment of the mendicant order," he bellowed.

To the sound of the quill scratching feverishly across parchment, Simon jerked his head up to see an evil grin spreading across the face of Palgrave. His blood ran cold. *Every fear he held deep in his soul had just been made manifest.*

"What evidence have you, sir?" called the magistrate.

Palgrave reached into a worn leather valise and produced five of the bloodiest, most gruesome illustrations he had stolen from the crates in Father Hardwicke's offices. He held the drawings high for all to see. "Evidence produced by the very hand of Simon McKensie, himself." He pushed his way forward and spread the illustrations across the magistrate's table, pointing to the signatures. He took a step back. "I further charge that a sacrilegious and unwarranted medical experiment was undertaken on a young woman at St. Bartholomew's yesterday noon. That experiment, a blood transfusion between a human being and a…a sheep," he sputtered in outrage, " by this…this heretic, resulted in the death of the young woman, MaryPryde Beckwith."

The crowd cried out in condemnation and jeers at Simon. The magistrate examined the drawings, one parchment after the other. Shaking his head imperceptibly at each successive illustration, the magistrate looked to Simon, and then looked at the drawings once more. He set them aside. Holding his hand up to subdue the rowdy onlookers, the magistrate called out once more to the assembly. "Is there anyone willing to offer testimony on the defendants behalf?"

"I will."

Simon craned his head toward the rear of the chamber to see who stood in his defense. Relief washed over him as he watched as Father Hardwicke, dressed in his most formal vestments, walk forward. The boisterous crowd fell silent at the priest's calm, dignified bearing, parting in silence to allow him passage to the front of the chamber.

"I will, sir," repeated Father Hardwicke as he stepped to the table.

The legs of the magistrate's chair scraped hollowly on the wooden planks in the now quiet room as he pulled closer to the table. He gave the priest his full attention. "Aye, Father. Proceed."

Father Hardwicke glanced to Simon, giving him an encouraging nod. "This young man possesses an extraordinary intellect. He is scientifically curious, tireless in his quest for knowledge, and willing to work more hours in a day than are possible to obtain that knowledge for the betterment of all."

As the crowd murmured amongst themselves considering the argument, Simon felt the small stirrings of hope.

Father Hardwicke continued. "I observed Dr. McKensie during the procedure yesterday. As Head Administrator of St. Bartholomew's, McKensie had my full warrant to conduct the experiment. The volunteer was cautioned that there could be no guarantees on the outcome and yet, she willingly gave her consent. I examined her throughout the day. Miss Beckwith was strong throughout the procedure, and gave no signs of ill health during her recovery. As to the illustrations, I do not believe that a full signature appears on any of the parchments, however, I can assert under oath that any scientific knowledge gained from such a procedure has advanced our knowledge of medicine at the hospital. For those reasons, I bear witness this day that Dr. Simon McKensie is *not* guilty of the crimes leveled against him."

The fickle crowd thundered its approval at the testimony given by Father Hardwicke, for an enthusiastic rebuttal was always highly entertaining. Father Hardwicke walked back to Catherine and took her hand protectively into his own. The magistrate silenced the assemblage, taking a moment to consider both sides of the issue. He looked through the illustrations once more. Simon felt his heart sink at the momentary expression of revulsion that crossed the magistrate's countenance.

The magistrate looked up, and then called to Simon. "Come forward."

The chains clanked dully on the floorboards as Simon made his way to the table. He could see the anguish in Catherine's eyes and it tore at his heart. He had never caused another such pain. *I should never have married her, for I have brought dishonor and scandal upon us.* He turned from her in his shame.

The magistrate stood to make his pronouncement. "I have looked at the evidence presented this day and heard the reasoning by both the accuser and the testimony offered upon the defendant's behalf. I understand and appreciate the pursuit of scientific knowledge as it benefits society as a whole, however, a young woman lies this day dead, a young woman who would be alive still had it not been for the medical intervention of the defendant."

Simon lowered his head. He knew what was to come.

"I have also examined the illustrations. And while it is yet to be determined if the signatures, the drawings, and the acts which these illustrations depict are attributable to the defendant, the charge of grave-robbing, exhumation, dissection and dismemberment is punishable by death by hanging." He paused. "Moreover, the charge of murder carries with it the punishment of death by hanging."

Simon held his breath. In the back of the room, Catherine clutched at Father Hardwicke, leaning against him for support.

The magistrate lifted his head and looked straight at Simon. "I believe the evidence presented on this day, 8 March, 1667, against Doctor Simon McKensie to be True Bills."

The crowd gasped. Father Hardwicke grabbed Catherine as she sagged at the knees.

"I therefore recommend that the defendant be remanded to Clink Prison. Trial will commence Friday, 11 March. Ten o'clock in the morning." At that, the magistrate stood and left the room.

In tears, Catherine pushed her way through the crowd to the front of the room. She reached out for Simon. A guard stepped in her path and restrained her. "Let me go," she cried, straining against the arms that held her back. "Let me go!"

Simon looked back to her in anguish as he was led away. "Send for the mayor!" he cried out. The guards yanked him through the wooden doors that led out to the street where a horse-drawn prison cart awaited. Catherine broke free from the guard and ran outside, watching them throw Simon unceremoniously into the back of the cart.

The gaunt man from the front of the room turned toward Catherine wearing a strange wooden plank on a leather strap hanging about his neck with holders for small inkpots and space for his parchment. He shoved several men away, dipping his quill into the pot. "Miss?" he shouted. "Miss, over 'ere, please!"

Catherine, threading her way through the crowd toward Simon, stopped when she realized he was yelling at her. "Who are you?" she cried, pushing through the shouting, shoving onlookers.

"Grimes, Miss. From the Gazette!" he shouted back as the crowd surrounded her. "Are ye Lady McKensie, the murderer's missus?"

Horrified, Catherine whirled away to see the driver slap the reins sharply against the horse's flanks. "Simon!" she cried, holding her hand high for him to see. "Simon!"

Realizing that the London Gazette had sent a scribe for Lady McKensie, the onlookers ran for her. They tore at her clothes and hair. They clawed at her handbag, grasping for any bit of her they could reach. Someone grabbed her hand and began to pull at her gold wedding ring. Catherine cried out, and slapped the dirt-encrusted hands away. Fighting her way through the crowd, Catherine ran out to the lane.

"Get on!" snarled the driver, flogging the horses harder. They snorted, straining against the bit, then reluctantly clopped forward, spewing dirt and dust in their wake.

Dazed, Catherine stood on the cobbles, helpless as to what to do. "I love you," Simon mouthed, as the swaying prison cart pulled away. Father Hardwick caught up to her. Ashen-faced, she turned to him as if to speak, and then Catherine fainted in his arms.

CHAPTER THIRTY-SIX

Bealeton House
St. James Parish, London
Tuesday, 8 March 1667
7:35 pm

Catherine leaned on the palm of one hand at the cookery's long serving table, idly shoving bits of meat on her plate from one side to the other. Unable to think any longer, she gazed at the whitewashed bricks of the coved ceiling, and then to the tidy row of copper pots hanging neatly on a custom iron rack from the largest to the smallest. Even the table had been carefully thought out. It could seat three, or thirty, depending on the size of the staff brought in for special occasions. Viola had planned every detail. With a start, Catherine realized how much she had missed her aunt, and how much she needed her now. It had been a very long day. She feared the night would prove much longer.

A faint, new moon seeping through the windows set high in the plastered walls bathed Catherine's troubled face in soft light. Gussie ladled a second plate from the pot, then set the plate down on the table next to a thick beeswax candle and wiped her eyes with the back of her hand. She sat heavily on the bench. "I canna' believe she's gone. I just canna' believe it" she said, shaking her head. "Aye'n a fine lass, she was. Such grand plans, an' all." Her eyes wet once more, Gussie looked to Catherine. She hesitated. "Ye dinna' think Simon had anything to do with it, do ye lassie?"

Catherine sat up. "No, I do not, Gussie," she said, firmly. "Though I cannot say exactly what did happen, I know with all my heart that Simon did not murder MaryPryde." Catherine set the fork down, unable to contemplate the unimaginable.

Concerned, Gussie moved the plate of fragrant rabbit stew closer to her. "Ye've nae touched yer food. Ye've got to eat, my lamb," she said, her voice a gentle rebuke.

Catherine took the fork back in hand. She tried a small bite, and then looked to the cook, tears beginning to stain her own cheeks. "I fear I've no appetite, Gussie," she said, wiping her own eyes.

Gussie narrowed her eyes. "I'd say it's yer worries for Simon that's got ye in knots, but the truth of it is, lassie… ye've nae had yer courses in two months." She paused a moment, smiling gently. "Tha' wee bairn'll make itself known by late summer, like as not." Gussie leveled a serious gaze. "I know yer worried, but ye've got to look after the both of ye, nae, Catherine."

Gussie rarely called her Catherine, and when she did, she meant business, for nothing escaped the cook's attention. "Oh, Gussie, I've never been so frightened in my life," Catherine breathed, tears streaming once more. "No one can know, at least not until we sort this out."

Gussie's practical nature took hold. "Aye, my lamb, I'll not speak of it t' a soul, so longs' as ye take good care." Gussie stood and gave Catherine an encouraging hug about the shoulders. "Archie's gone to fetch Charles and the mayor. I expect they'll travel through the night, and on the morrow, the three of ye'll put yer 'eads together an' think of something, like as not," she said, firmly. "Nae, it's late. Finish yer stew, an' go on up to bed. Ye'll be needin' yer sleep to think clearly as ye can in the mornin'."

For the first time in that very long day, Catherine managed a wan smile. "Aye, Gussie, I will, indeed."

Up in the quiet of her third floor chamber, Catherine sat in the chair by the front window and looked out to the stars sparkling in the dark skies over the West End. Not knowing where Simon was or if he was safe was agonizing in the extreme. She drew her knees to her chest to quell the sickening knot that was forming in the pit of her stomach. Catherine dropped her head and cried, as exhaustion and worry at last overwhelmed.

∽∾∽

Simon gingerly laid his aching head back against the stone walls of the basement in Clink prison. The guard had dragged him down the steps and thrown him straight into a cramped cell at the bottom, slamming the thick iron bars shut with a resounding clank. Off balance, Simon tripped over the shackles at his ankles and fell, cracking his forehead on the cold stone floor. When he came to, disoriented and bloodied, he could not say how long he had been in the cell. In the pitch black, something small and furry skittered over his hand. He cried out, pulling his hand back in revulsion.

"Oi!" growled a deep voice near the bars.

"My…my apologies. It's just that it's dark, and I'm not entirely sure where I am."

A sharp, scratch as flint was struck to tinderbox, then a feeble candleflame illuminated the shadowy chamber. The other cells were empty. Simon was alone in the dank, foul-smelling basement. He shivered, though he could not say for sure it was the freezing air that leeched in through the cracks, or the sinister foreboding he felt rising in the pit of his stomach. His cell was bare, save a soiled chamber pot in the corner. The dirt floor smelled of vomit. A rat, stretching on its hind legs to climb the wall, turned two glowing, pink eyes toward the light, momentarily blinding itself in its glare. Simon scrambled from the rodent. "Vile creature!" he blurted, recoiling against the thick iron bars.

The guard laughed at his retreat. "Aye, them cursed vermin'll nibble at yer ears, yer feet, yer fingers—whatever they kin' find in th' dark."

Simon thought he would be sick.

"Light scares 'em off, though," he drawled, with the taunting air of a resourceful, underpaid man anxious for an extra bit of scratch.

"Light?"

"If ye've coin enough, a' course," he tempted. "A bit of straw to sleep on… A gobbet to eat, too, if ye've a mind to it."

The pounding in Simon's head confused him. "I beg your pardon, sir. What exactly are you saying?"

"Candle's two penny. Straw t' lay yer 'ead on, five p. Nae if ye've a mind t' a meal while yer 'ere, why, that'll be ten. *Each.*" The guard scratched his filthy, stubbled chin. "An' if ye'd like them chains off, why that'll be more, a' course," he leered, with an evil grin.

Simon reached into his pockets for his leather pouch. Both pockets were empty. "I…I don't seem to have…" He tried the pocket at his chest. "I seem to have, ah' lost my… " He looked up to the guard. "It's missing. My coin pouch is missing."

The guard spit on the ground, unfazed. "Aye. Tha'll 'appen' round 'ere." He blew out the candle. "Mind th' rats," he grunted, as he trudged up the stone steps. A key rattled. The door opened a crack to a star-filled sky, and then banged shut again, leaving Simon alone in the darkness. *He wondered if he'd ever see the stars again.* Outside, the lock rattled once more and then, silence.

CHAPTER THIRTY-SEVEN

Bealeton House
St. James Parish, London
Wednesday, 9 March 1667
8:34 am

After a fitful night of sleep, Catherine awoke to a commotion in the courtyard beneath her third floor suite. She sighed and threw back the covers. Sleep was hopeless. She walked to the window and parted the velvet window hangings that still carried the thick scent of smoke these many months after the fire. Catherine looked down upon the sight of the abbey carriage and two kitchen carts pulling into the courtyard. More carts would follow in the days to come, she knew, for Aunt Viola and the mayor had returned, bringing with them staff and provisions enough to fill the house to the brim. Despite her troubles, Catherine managed a smile. The house would churn with activity and formality once again. Gone would be the comfortable dinners with Gussie and Archie in the kitchen, and the private, quiet nights spent before the fire with Simon. *Simon.* The nauseous feeling in her stomach returned ten-fold. She sank to the chair at the thought. He was alone. In prison. For murder. For once, she was at a complete loss. She missed her father more than ever. He always knew the right course to take. A knock at the door brought her attentions back to the commotion outside.

Gussie bustled in. "Good morning, lassie. Yer aunt and the mayor have returned. Let's get ye dressed. They're wantin' to speak with ye."

"Thank you, Gussie," Catherine said, rising quickly.

"An' they'll speak t' ye *after* the mornin' meal," said Gussie, pulling a day gown from the armoire with a very firm hand.

Catherine looked at Gussie, and the determined set to her face, an expression she knew meant no argument. "Aye."

❦

The mayor took a seat at the head of the table in the dining room. Though he looked well rested and hale after his three months confinement at the abbey, his face betrayed a noticeable concern as he caught up with the London news in the Gazette handbill. Though he would not speak to it, along with Simon's likeness, there was a large headline blaring news of the experiment and the death of MaryPryde. Viola and Charles, sitting to either side of the mayor, looked equally anxious. An Abbey maid served breakfast in the hushed room.

"Thank you, Jemma," the mayor smiled.

The mayor carefully folded the handbill over, and then set it beneath his plate as Catherine joined them at the table. Jemma set a large plate of eggs and sausages with currants before her. Catherine was about to protest the generous serving, but the maid stopped her short.

"From Gussie, Milady."

Catherine nodded in surrender, realizing that she was, in fact, ravenous. She took a bite, and then looked across the table to the faces she loved the most in this world, unspeakably grateful. "Thank you all so much for coming," she said, tears filling her eyes.

"I am afraid I still do not quite understand all that has transpired," said the mayor. "Can you explain exactly what happened?"

As Catherine related the experiment and its tragic outcome, Viola murmured in dismay. Charles, dipping his quill repeatedly in an inkpot, took copious notes in his ledger.

When she finished, the mayor was silent for a moment as he considered the facts. Charles set his quill on the table and looked to Catherine. "If I may, I believe you and I should pay an immediate visit to the prison. Having spent these months at the Inns of Court, I have been privy to certain, ah' information that might be of help."

"What sort of information, Charles?" asked Catherine, tucking into the fresh eggs.

Charles furrowed his brow, looking first to the ladies, then back to the mayor, unsure as to whether he should speak frankly.

"Restraint, while admirable, Charles, is quite futile under the circumstances," said Viola, her tone crisp and to the point. "I think it best to speak out."

Charles and Catherine exchanged a surprised glance. Since her marriage to the mayor, their dithering aunt had somehow become an unexpected force of both logic and practicality.

Charles took a deep breath. "Simon is being held in Clink prison. In other circumstances, of course, he would have been taken to either Newgate or Old Bailey, but the fire has destroyed them both. Either one would have been preferable, however, for Clink is the most notorious of the three, being run by unscrupulous guards and a cruel warden."

Both Catherine and Viola visibly blanched. The mayor, looking as though he might wish to silence Charles, nodded instead. "Go on."

"There are certain advantages to be had, however." He hesitated to suggest an unsavory course. "Because the guards are underpaid, if they are paid at all, they are amenable to... certain temptations."

"I beg your pardon?" asked Catherine, desperate for any hope to be had.

"They can be...ah, negotiated with," said Charles. He glanced to the mayor.

"What does that mean?" Catherine asked once more.

"They can be bribed for better treatment," interrupted Viola. "Charles and Catherine, go at once to the solicitor. Have him advance you any amount Charles believes will help Simon."

She had another thought. "Cecil, perhaps you could use your influence to secure an appointment with the king?"

Jemma, clearing the plates, glanced toward Viola. A momentary flash of condemnation crossed her face as she left the room. Catherine caught the disapproving glance. *The old man in the street. MaryPryde. A maid in her own house.*

"Would that be right?" whispered Catherine, embarrassed. "Is that not an unjust advantage?"

"Why on earth would it not be right?" asked Viola, incredulous. "Why, the very idea."

"I understand, my dear," said the mayor. "I often wonder myself if having 'the King's ear,' so to speak, is unjust, since so many do not possess the same opportunity."

"You would wish Simon suffer needlessly, when we might petition for royal pardon? "We have but three days, Catherine," said Viola, shaking her head at the very thought. "There is no time to debate the point."

"One set of laws for those with means, another for those without," Catherine whispered, remembering the first time she met MaryPryde. "I...I do not know the right course."

Charles spoke up. "Your point is well taken, however, I ask only this. Do you believe Simon is guilty? Of murder? Catherine, they will *hang* him."

A sudden clarity came over Catherine. "No. I do not!"

"Then, my dear..." said the mayor, gently, "...we must use all means available."

Her thoughts cleared in an instant. "You are right, of course—we must pursue all avenues!" With dismay, she sat up, remembering the evening at Whitehall. "But the king is not in residence. He has traveled to Malmesbury. It is said he will not return for several weeks."

Charles looked to Cecil. "Perhaps we might secure an audience with the Duke of York to intervene on Simon's behalf?"

"Aye, lad, I'm afraid the Duke is currently at sea refortifying the southern coast," he said, setting his hand to the newspaper.

They all fell into silent contemplations. Every course they had considered led to an insurmountable obstacle. Charles looked back at his notes, as if there were something he had missed, something, anything that might help.

The formless sense of dread, the desperate helplessness that had tormented Catherine from the moment the guards appeared in the administration offices suddenly dissipated. *She had influential friends of her own.*

CHAPTER THIRTY-EIGHT

"I AM WRAPPED IN DISMAL THINKING"
~ WILLIAM SHAKESPEARE

Clink Prison
Southwark, London
Wednesday, 9 March 1667
11:48 am

Simon thought he might well go mad. Sleep eluded him through the long, harrowing night, as he weighed every decision, every course, every moment of the experiment. How could he have been so certain? How could he have so carelessly intervened in the life of another? What had he done? He nearly broke down contemplating the sadness—and the unknown science—of it all. Was it the blood that took her life? Did the cells not join issue? Was there a poisoning between the two fluids? The tormented thoughts made his head ache beyond reason. The fallow line between day and night, between right and wrong, between sanity and madness, was splintering by the hour. Nothing made sense. Would that he could have performed a *post mortem* on MaryPryde. Surely the logic and scientific observation of the procedure would have offered some measure of relief to the profound desolation he felt. He shivered in the cold air that seeped into the cellar from the crack under the door, though, in truth, he was grateful there was a crack, for it was the only way he could distinguish day from night. He shifted his position on the hard dirt and drew his tunics closer to ward off both the cold air and the unceasing dread that surrounded him.

A sudden, frigid blast of wind sent leaves and dirt swirling down the steps as the door opened, then banged shut once more. Simon could hear footsteps scuffling toward him, though in the pale light, he could not see it was the guard until the man stood outside the cell banging on the bars with his wooden truncheon. "On yer feet," the man growled. Simon rose awkwardly, the shackles digging into his ankles. The guard rattled a key in the lock, hollowly wrenching it hard it to the right. Simon watched as the creaking iron bars swung wide, unsure as to what to do. "Come on, then."

Still shackled, Simon followed the guard up the steps as best he could, then across a small courtyard toward another building. Two people stood with their backs to him in the wide, austere quadrangle. *He knew her instantly.* "Catherine," he cried out.

Whirling about, Catherine raced to Simon. They stood, clinging to one another as one would to a mighty oak in a gathering storm. "I'm frightened, Simon," whispered Catherine.

"I know, my darling. I am, too."

Simon held her in his arms as long as he could, before Charles stepped to them, setting his hand on Simon's shoulder. "Please forgive me, but I must ask. Besides Father Hardwicke and the mayor, can you think of anyone else who might testify on your behalf?"

For long a moment, Simon could not think clearly. I…I do not believe there is…" He looked to Catherine in confusion. The overwhelming sadness in her eyes nearly broke his heart.

Catherine took his hands into hers and looked up to him. "I intend to speak to Lady Wilbraham, perhaps she will appeal to the Countess of Castlemaine."

The Countess of Castlemaine. Suddenly the fog in his memory cleared. "Yes! Yes, there is someone who might stand to my defense. The king's chemyst, Sir Robert Boyle. He has heard of my efforts in Wells and has invited me to speak at Oxford. Charles, you will find him up at Gresham."

"Aye, I shall call upon him today," said Charles, much

heartened by Simon's acquaintance with the famous physick. "Well done, Simon."

With the barest hint of hope rising, Simon reached for Catherine. He took her into his arms for as long as he dared, stroking her hair, inhaling the soft scent of her skin, memorizing every inch of her. He closed his eyes to the grim reality he faced. How he missed her. *How he desperately needed her.* He felt her slip a small but heavy packet into the pocket of his tunics.

"Enough!" cried the guard, cracking Simon across the back with his truncheon.

Simon was knocked to the ground from the force of the blow. He lay on the stones, writhing in pain.

"There is no need to strike him!" Catherine cried out.

"Come, Catherine!" Charles drew Catherine away, desperately entreating her to remain silent.

The guard pulled Simon from the ground and turned to lead him toward another set of stairs at the rear of the yard.

"I shall come again tomorrow," she cried out, breaking free from Charle's grasp.

"Nae, ye won't," grunted the guard, as he struggled to keep Simon upright in the ankle chains. "One visit," he leered back at her. "Rules is rules, even fer such a fine lady as yerself." An evil grin spread across his face.

Desperate for Simon's safety, she stopped short in the courtyard and turned to Charles in disbelief. "How can this be happening?" she whispered.

Climbing the narrow wooden staircase, Simon jerked from the guard's grasp for one last look back. "I…I'm sorry, Catherine," he whispered. "I'm sorry." He turned from the pain he could see in her face. He had caused it. *He could not bear it.*

"Quiet!" The guard kicked a door open at the top of the stairs, and shoved Simon inside. "Ye've been paid fer."

"I've been what?"

The guard dragged him down a dim, narrow passageway.

As he passed each foreboding cell, a pair of eyes followed him, though to a man, the prisoners were silent. "Yer people have made, ah'…shall we say, a 'contribution' towards yer well-bein'." He grinned and rattled several heavy coins in his pocket. "Yer t' 'ave two meals a day, an' ye'll sleep here until yer trial." The guard unlocked the irons to an austere cell. "Tis our finest chamber," he said, affecting an upper crust accent. "I do hope ye'll find it right comfortable," he leered, before removing the shackles at Simon's feet. The heavy chains clanked across the floorboards as the guard trudged out, locking the iron bars behind him.

Simon stood alone, taking stock of the cramped, spare billet. A chamber pot sat beneath a small, barred window. A bucket of water stood next to it. On the window's thick, stone sill sat a single candle, flint and tinderbox. A layer of straw had been tossed on the wooden floorboards for a pallet, although how long it had been there, he could not say. A threadbare blanket was thrown in a heap upon the straw. There were no other luxuries. Through the bars across the passageway, he could see an unfortunate lump of a man curled up on a bare floor with nothing but a chamber pot in his cell. The man groaned and shifted his weight, but did not awaken.

Simon sighed, and then sat down on the straw contemplating his dismal fate. He looked down at his raw, stinging ankles. The shackles had left dark red trails of blood that dripped from his feet onto the straw. He sat down and ripped several strips from his outer tunic, and then tied the fabric around the wounds to staunch the flow. Something heavy in his pocket hit the floorboards. Turning to face the wall, he pulled the leather packet out, untied the laces and looked inside. *Catherine had slipped him coins.* It was a complete mystery how she knew these things, yet, nothing she did surprised him. Daring not to breathe, he slid the packet under the straw, quickly glancing to the lump across the way. The man was still asleep. Exhaling a sigh of relief, Simon leaned against the bars, then looked down to see dark, red blood seeping through the heavy cotton strips. *The blood. MaryPryde. Death by hanging.* For the very first time in his life, Simon was scared. He exhaled and sank to the straw, then closed his eyes and prayed for sleep.

CHAPTER THIRTY-NINE

Creaking rafters in the loft above the barn shook Oswold awake as the door was thrown wide, sending flurries of hay and draff from the stored wheat into his eyes and mouth. Spitting softly, he shifted the hay from a crack in the floorboards and looked down to the stable below. He drew a sharp breath. His father stood just below the loft unharnessing the plow horse. A small piece of hay tickled his nose. Stifling a sneeze, his thoughts were a jumble. *How long have I slept?*

The horse snorted, jerking its head, as the leathers were unhooked. "Aye, Pen, old gal, " soothed Josiah Haggett, patting the horse on the withers. The horse whinnied and drew its leg up. Josiah looked at the horse with concern. "Easy, easy… I know it hurts. Me leg 'urts, too." Josiah chuckled to himself. "You an' me, Penderal, why we're gittin' old as the hills."

Through the crack, Oswold watched as Josiah clicked his teeth and stroked the horse's mane with thick, calloused hands. "Aye, another year or two, why we'll both be set out t' pasture."

Oswold's heart went soft. His father was getting old. Too old to farm from sunup to sundown, but the farm was pledged against Oswold's medical training. With his mother dead of the plague and no brothers or sisters, there was no one else to work the clover fields and no money left to pay for extra help. Oswold was tormented by the plight he found himself in. *His charge against Palgrave would bring his father to ruin.* And yet, if he kept the crime to himself, Doctor McKensie would be convicted, that he knew. *The wrong man would hang.* He watched his father groom the horse. Methodical and gentle in his ways, his father and the horse were two souls in perfect accord. With everything in such upheaval, the familiar routine soothed Oswold's troubled thoughts.

Josiah set the brushes in a wooden box, and then placed the box neatly on a nearby shelf. "Aye Penders ol' gal, tha's it for today." He opened the door to the nearest stall and gave the horse a friendly pat on the rump. The horse walked straight to the oats. Oswold felt a rumble in his own stomach. He was hungry. He knew he should go into the house, though he dared not face his father with the knowledge that the farm would be lost. His stomach rumbled again. He would steal into the house for food after his father fell asleep. One more night in the barn, one more night of sleep would do them both good. *He would tell his father in the morning.*

CHAPTER FORTY

"LAY THIS UNTO YOUR BREAST. OLD FRIENDS LIKE
OLD SWORDS, STILL ARE TRUSTED BEST"
~ JOHN WEBSTER, 1637

Whitehall Palace
Private Apartments
Wednesday, 9 March 1667
7:00pm

The Countess of Castlemaine sat at her dressing table wincing under the laborious attentions of a young maid as the girl twined a red ribbon through the dark curls of her sweeping updo. A knock at the door startled them both.

"Yes?" called the countess, pushing the maid's hands away. "That hurts! Leave it," she said, exasperated. "Just leave it..." The maid tied off the ribbon and, trembling, reached for an emerald necklace that lay atop a careless pile of jewels. The countess seized the necklace and flung it back onto the pile. "No, the rubies," she said, irritated at the dull-witted maid's ineptitude. The countess lifted the necklace toward the firelight to admire the sparkling reflections in its crimson facets.

The maid took the necklace and fastened it around the countess's neck. Then, with tentative hands, the girl reached for the comb once more. "Shall I finish?" she whispered. The countess lifted her eyes to the heavens, praying for restraint as her lady-in-waiting, Lady Compton, stepped into the room.

"Yes?"

"The Ladies Wilbraham and McKensie, and Mrs. Dillworth wish to speak with you, Countess."

"'Tis an early hour, but show them in." The countess looked

up to the maid still standing behind her, pearl-handled comb in hand. "Are you still here?"

The maid blushed and skittered away as Lady Compton led the guests into the chamber. The countess rose from the dressing table, glad to be free of the maid's clumsy attentions. She gestured across the room to a sitting area before the fire. "Lovely to see you! Please… please, sit," said the countess, taking her place at the center of a rose-embroidered settee. "Shall we have champagne?" she said, merrily. The countess took a moment to arrange her voluminous skirts, and then looked at the three solemn faces. She faced the three women, suddenly curious. "Perhaps this is not the time," she said softly. "What brings you to my salon at this early hour?"

Elizabeth glanced to Catherine who nodded her assent. "We wish to make an appeal to the King."

The countess raised her eyebrows. "Go on."

Setting her hand to Catherine's shoulder, Pippa interrupted. "This is Lady Catherine McKensie—perhaps you recall an introduction at your salon last Saturday."

"Perhaps. It was a rather bungled evening," she said, dryly.

Pippa glanced to Elizabeth, and then continued. "Her husband has met with a certain misfortune."

The countess was quiet for a moment. "Husband," she mused, staring down at her bejeweled fingers. The countess sighed, as she played with the large ruby ring on her right hand, twisting it first to the right and then to the left. "A husband is a luxury I fear I'll not see."

Pippa opened her mouth to reassure the countess, but was stopped by a cautionary hand on her arm. "Let her speak," whispered Elizabeth. Pippa fell silent.

In the warmth of the sumptuous, feminine chamber, a strange air of melancholy seemed to befall the countess. Catherine looked from Elizabeth to Pippa, unsure of the unexpected turn in the conversation.

"Thus wisher wants their will, and that they will do crave…" murmured the countess, holding her hand up to admire the ruby. "A wisher I am, indeed, and my will I do crave, but as Master Shakespeare hath foretold, ne'er shall it be."

"Countess? Are you quite well?" asked Pippa, her brows knitted in concern.

Paying no attention to her, the countess looked to the ladies with a dawning realization. "I have borne him two children, and yet, *she* wears his ring. She does nothing, and gives nothing. She sacrifices nothing save her days, which she devotes from sunrise to sunset in prayer." She twisted the ring on her finger. "I *have* nothing, you see, but my wits, my temper…and my womb." She stared at herself in the mirror from across the room and set a gentle hand upon the necklace. "And my jewels." She faced the threesome with a strange, soft smile. "'Tis an unending toil to bewitch a king. Yet, if I do not, if I grow old, or ill or tired, I am most easily replaced by the next 'pretty, witty Nell' from the king's merry playhouse." She stared at Catherine, the air thick with sudden emotion. "You are a fortunate woman, Lady McKensie."

The ladies fell silent at the unsettling glimpse of fragility from the customarily gay and witty countess. The countess sighed. "There are days when one wonders why they were placed on this earth, are there not?"

Discomfited in the extreme by self-reflection, Pippa stepped in to draw the conversation back. "Countess, if…if we might speak of her husband? You see, he has been arrested and charged with murder."

The countess tilted her head in thought. She looked to Catherine with interest. "Your husband is the physick, Simon McKensie?"

"He is, Countess," said Catherine. "And as of two days ago…"

"You need not go on," interrupted the Countess, raising a hand. "I am aware of your husband's plight. Robert Boyle has this day delivered a letter with an entreaty to the king on your husband's behalf."

Catherine exhaled with relief.

"We have come to ask you to do the same, Countess," said Elizabeth.

Catherine leaned toward the countess, her voice low and urgent. "You must understand that there was no malice on my husband's part. His only intention was scientific inquiry," she said. "MaryPryde Beckwith was in good health and constitution in the hours after the experiment and there is no explanation for her death, except to say that it *was* indeed an experiment. It was fully explained to MaryPryde that there were no guarantees of her safety. She wished to participate nonetheless." Catherine wiped a tear. "He is to be tried for murder in but hours, not days, Countess. We have no time to mount an earnest defense. Our only hope of reprieve may be a pardon from the king,"

"We do not wish to trade unduly upon our friendship, Countess, but time has created an urgency," said Pippa.

The countess looked troubled. "The king has taken refuge at Malmesbury—a full three day's ride from London. I do not expect—nor do I wish—him to return in less that a fortnight, though were he closer he might be prevailed upon in time."

The ladies fell silent as Elizabeth turned her practical mind to the problem. She suddenly turned to the countess. "The king travels with an entire royal entourage, does he not?"

Catherine caught her meaning. "A messenger riding alone through the night might cover the distance in far less time?"

"Yes!" cried Pippa. "A single rider would indeed travel faster!"

Elizabeth caught the countess's hands in her own. "Will you help Lady McKensie?"

"I beg of you, Countess," said Catherine, the slight waver in her voice betraying an abject fear.

In that moment, in the midst of the gilt and rose-hued opulence of her royal apartments, the beautiful, bewitching Barbara Villiers, Countess of Castlemaine, felt the deep ache of unrelenting loneliness. Unlike these women, she had no real friends. In all truth, fair-spoken ladies in waiting surrounded her, and at her fingertips were a coterie of servants to satisfy her every pleasure, but such loyalties were bound in great measure by cunning ambitions. *The true bonds of friendship could not, nae, would not flourish in such company.* She longed for the king more than she would allow, yet, she would not crawl upon her knees in repentance. He had humiliated *her. With an actress.* Were she prone to self-reflection, she would have to admit that she herself humiliated the queen each day in much the same fashion, but such wisdom was not a gift she possessed. She lived by her wits. And, she knew well the terms. She would not beg him to return. A sudden thought struck. *Perhaps he was longing for her.* Perhaps a letter scented with her earthy, bergamot fragrance would evoke such lustful, sensual, *sinful* memories that would fell him to his knees with desire. Perhaps he would come back begging *her* forgiveness. She arched her brow. *Yes, a letter.* Her foul mood brightened considerably. "Lady Compton, bring me parchment and quill—and send for Stokes. He is the fastest among the messengers." She smiled at Catherine. "Tell him he is to ride immediately."

CHAPTER FORTY-ONE

"THOUGH LUST DO MASQUE IN NE'ER SO STRANGE
DISGUISES, SHE'S OFT FOUND WITTY, BUT IS NEVER WISE"
~ JOHN WEBSTER, 1661

Berkshire Forest
Thursday, 10 March 1667
2:07 am

Royal Messenger Tobias Stokes thundered through the murky woodlands of Berkshire deep in the night, charging to the west toward Wiltshire from London. He had been summoned abruptly from his supper, and his stomach was rumbling, though he dared not stop, not even for a handful of field greens that grew wild on the forest floor. The countess had chosen him personally for his swiftness and like all who served at the pleasure of the king and court, Stokes had a right and proper fear of the woman's volcanic temperament.

Lanterns dangling from his saddlebags cast strange shadows upon the well-traveled path as he urged his horse onward through the darkness. The hours raced by. Passing from forest to field, the road at last leveled straight and true, and as he galloped westward, his thoughts began to drift. Holding the reins comfortably in his left hand, he raised his right hand and inhaled deeply. The calloused skin on his fingers held a faint, earthy scent that excited him no end. That scent played heavily upon his mind, for the beautiful Countess of Castlemaine knew him very well—and not just for his speed in the saddle.

There had been yet another 'disaccord' between the countess and the king at Hampton Court. In a fiery rage, the countess had stormed out to the stables intending to ride back to London alone, though she confessed to being unsure of the way. Tobias, newly promoted to the king's stables, feared for the horse, and had offered his services as escort on her ride, although something, a momentary flash in her violet-hued eyes made him think she was not as unaccustomed to the path as she vouchsafed.

He had accompanied her deep into the forest surrounding the palace. As they rode past a waterfall tucked into a fern-laden brae, she claimed a thirst and dismounted, wrenching an ankle as she set foot to earth. In her agony, she reached for his grasp. Against his better judgment, for the royal retribution would surely be swift and merciless, Tobias swung her into his arms and carried her toward a mossy log that had fallen at the side of the stream. To the deafening sound of water eddying over the rocks, he held the countess close to his chest as he walked, catching the scent of her perfume. The sensual fragrance lingered long in his memory, for the earthy, bergamot scent bore a faint note of citrus that well mingled with the forest around them. Her scent was intoxicating. The countess sat on the edge of the log rubbing her ankle. She looked up at him with a tantalizing smile that stirred his senses. He stood his ground until he could take it no more. Casting off the cry of restraint in his soul, Tobias took her into his arms. The kiss was deep and intense. He could not keep his hands from her. She was indeed, as proclaimed by all who met her, bewitching. This he knew, for Tobias himself had in that moment fallen under her spell. When at last, he came to his better senses, Tobias pulled from her grasp. What in God's name had he done? They had gathered their things, remounted and ridden back to the castle with nary a word spoken between them. The brief encounter lay dormant, willfully forgotten in his memory until this night when he had been summoned by the countess to deliver two letters to the king.

In the pale light of a waxing moon, Tobias reached down and pulled the letters from his saddlebag. Holding tight to the fragrant letter, he tucked the other back into the bag and closed the flap. He closed his eyes and inhaled deeply of the seductive perfume, then Tobias bent toward the saddle, curled his lips into a sly grin, and kicked the horse hard. The powerful thoroughbred surged forward in the darkness, as he savored the tantalizing memories all the way to Malmesbury House.

CHAPTER FORTY-TWO

Clink Prison
Southwark, London
Thursday, 10 March 1667
9:34 am

"re," growled yet another bewhiskered, foul-smelling guard, clanking a ladle through the iron bars. Simon lifted a wooden bowl to catch the clump of gray mush that fell into it. A chunk of doughy bread was dropped on top. Outside, horizontal sheets of rain spattered on the window glass, the filthy water surging through a wide gap in the wooden frame. Water poured down the wall into his cell and collected in a low spot next to the straw pallet. Shivering against the cold that leached through the stones, Simon was miserable in the extreme. Outside, the ceaseless pounding of a mallet upon nails reverberated through his troubled, aching head. The guard listened for a moment, then cocked an eyebrow at Simon and grinned. "Oi. Thas fer you." He winked and shuffled away. Simon's blood ran cold.

A low moan in the cell across from Simon interrupted his moribund thoughts. He glanced through the bars to see the lump of a man still lying on the floor in a puddle of rainwater. Another groan. Concerned, Simon looked closer. The man was shaking, desperate to catch his breath.

"Sir?" Simon called out. There was no answer.

The man groaned once more, then rolled over, panting. Simon could see sweat beads dripping from the man's face. "Guard!" shouted Simon, rising in his cell. "Guard!" he shouted through the bars.

"Quiet!" the guard yelled from the other end of the hall, banging his ladle on the irons of the closest cell.

"Please, this man is very ill."

The guard walked back. "An' what concern is it t' ye?" he said, glancing to the suffering man with all the curiosity of one who could not have cared less.

"I am a physick. This man has had nothing to eat since I have been here. He needs more food. He needs water and blankets or he will die!"

The man moaned once more, shivering in the water that had collected on the floor.

Simon shrugged off his outer tunic and shoved it through the bars. "Here. Give him this. He is very cold."

The guard took the tunic in hand and examined it. "So am I," he said, wrapping the tunic around his shoulders. "So am I." The guard walked back down the row, clanking his ladle on every cell door, just for spite.

"Wait…" shouted Simon, incredulous.

"Quiet!" the guard yelled. "Or ye'll go wi'out, jus' like 'im."

Simon was astonished at the cruelty. He glanced back to the man, and then pulled his water bucket over to the bars. "Can you come any closer?" he whispered.

The man dragged himself over toward Simon.

"What is your name?" asked Simon.

"John. Me name's John," he said, shivering. He had no wish to rile the guard further.

Simon lifted a ladle from the water bucket and slid it as best he could across the narrow passageway. He nodded. "Drink as much as you can."

"Thank ye," said John, grateful for a rare moment of kindness. John reached for the ladle with shaking hands, splashing water over the side. "My apologies, t' ye."

Simon slid him the loaf of bread, then stuffed his blanket through the bars, throwing it as far as he could. John grabbed hold of the corner and pulled it into his cell. "Wrap that around you," whispered Simon.

Still shaking, John crawled back to the corner and wrapped himself in the blanket. He took a bite of the bread, and then gave Simon a wan smile. "Thank ye, sir. Grateful t' ye.'"

Simon glanced to the window. Though the rain had stopped, the incessant hammering had not. He shuddered, trying to push from his mind the immense crowd that would gather in the quadrangle in less that twenty-four hours to watch him hang should he not mount a convincing defense. He looked through the rusting bars over to John, lying quiet in his misery. The hammering stopped. Simon closed his eyes in silent prayer. He knew the noose was waiting. *For him.* Simon looked to his pallet, and then sighed. Reaching beneath the straw, Simon pulled the leather pouch from its hiding place. He held the coins in his hand for a moment. Then, Simon leaned over to the bars. "Here," he whispered to John. Simon skidded the pouch across the floorboards. It slid through the bars and came to a rest at John's feet. "That will be more use to you than it will to me."

∞

Thursday, 10 March 1667
12:54 pm

Catherine wandered through Bealeton House, unable to concentrate, unable to think, unable to do much of anything except worry. She felt very much like the caged crickets Charles kept when he was young. Viola had taken to her bed and the mayor was out with Charles and the chymist, Robert Boyle, attempting to formulate a sound defense for the trial. The house was quiet, save the ticking of the French clock on the mantle above the fireplace. A cold shiver ran through Catherine's blood each time she glanced at it. *Less than twenty-four hours.* She paced anew. *They will hang him, Catherine.* Nothing made sense, and yet, she thought, there was something she must have missed. *A plus B always equals C.* The silence in the house was unnerving. She felt incapable of forming even a coherent sentence. *A plus B...* She thought of the experiment. Of Simon's careful preparations. Of MaryPryde and Father Hardwicke's presence that day. She felt a small twinge in her side and took a seat before the fire in the gathering room to rest. *The baby.* With all that was happening, she hadn't taken the time to consider anything except Simon. *What if she and the baby were left alone?* She shuddered, and then forcibly put the thought from her mind. She would cope with anything that came her way. *That she knew.* If nothing else, the last two years of her life had taught her that, but she refused to think of it. Gussie swept into the room, chasing the melancholy thoughts away.

"Thought ye'd like a bit of a natter, my lamb," said Gussie, setting a small tray of food on the hearth. "Ye promised me."

Catherine looked at the small loaf of bread and several generous wedges of Stilton. "I actually am quite peckish, Gussie."

"That's m' girl." Gussie stepped back, tripping slightly on the edge of the tapestry rug. "Clumsy of me," she smiled, straightening the rug with her foot.

Clumsy. Catherine sat up straight with a sudden thought of the medical students observing in the dissectory. A clumsy young man had stumbled from the stand after pushing his way through the students to help Simon. *What was his name?* In his sympathy for the young man's embarrassment, Simon had asked him to assist. Simon had even asked him to stay through the evening hours. *He was there that night!* Catherine jumped from the chair. "Gussie, I've got to go to the hospital!"

Alarmed, Gussie cried out. "Whatever for? Are ye all right?"

Catherine realized what she had said. "No, I have misspoken. I am fine, Gussie, but there was a student with MaryPryde that night. I have got to speak with him. Perhaps he saw something!"

"Will ye nae wait for Charles?"

"Charles did not say when he would return, and no, I cannot wait, Gussie. There is no time," said Catherine. She took another bite of cheese, and then wrapped the rest in the linen napkin. "I'll *not* wait." She put the bread and cheese in her pocket, fixing Gussie with a steady gaze.

Gussie shoulders slumped. "I'll tell Fitch to rig the carriage," she said, knowing she was overmatched. "I'll fix ye a packet—an' tell yer aunt when she wakes, as well" she sighed, looking for all the world as though she'd rather not.

⁓

Catherine stood with Gussie watching Fitch struggle with the carriage riggings. "My apologies, Milady. One of them irons is broke, an' it's nae holdin' the evener. If ye kin wait, I'll have it fixed in a tick."

Too worried to wait for Fitch to repair the broken iron, Catherine made a decision. She dared not glance to Gussie. "Please saddle Ganymeade, will you, Mr. Fitch?"

"Nae!" breathed Gussie. "Ye canna ride, Catherine!"

Catherine closed her eyes, thinking desperately of the baby she carried, and then looked at the watch hanging on a chain around her neck. Twenty hours remained until the trial. "I'll *not* lose Simon," she said, with a determined set to her chin. That determination wavered. "I cannot, Gussie," she whispered. "If something should happen while riding, the consequence will be mine alone." A single tear fell down her cheek. "And I alone shall have to accept that consequence."

Gussie set her hand to her lips, quelling her horror at the decision laid before Catherine. "Oh, lassie. 'Tis a choice King Solomon himself could nae make."

"You are going to make *me* cry, Gussie," Catherine said, her voice cracking with emotion. "But I have to think of Simon first." The tears flooded her eyes as she hugged the cook. "You do understand, do you not?"

"Aye, lassie," whispered Gussie, her own tears falling freely. "I would choose the same."

"Thank you, Gussie," said Catherine, her voice soft with the love she felt for the older woman.

"Are ye sure, Milady?" asked Fitch, as he saddled her horse in the stableyard. He looked to Gussie's tear-stained face. "Can ye nae wait for Master Charles?" he asked, suddenly concerned, although he could not say why. "I'd be happy t' drive ye m'self, though like I said, won't take but a tick to fix the riggin's."

"No, Mr. Fitch, thank you, but I'll not wait another moment."

Fitch lifted her into the saddle, and then gave the horse a solid pat on the rump. "Then, God be with ye, Milady."

"Thank you, Mr. Fitch," Catherine called back, as she wheeled her mount toward St. Bartholomew's.

Thursday, 10 March 1667
3:54 pm

Father Hardwicke sat at his desk in the hospital administration office, writing a defense of the lad he admired more than any student he had ever trained at St. Bartholomew's. He stared at the blank parchment, unable to order his thoughts, as though he still could not understand exactly what had transpired over the last three days. Angry shouts echoing down the hall caught his attention.

"You are not allowed back 'ere!"

"Let me pass, please!"

The priest recognized the voice of the registrar, but he did not recognize the woman. He did not have to wait long. The door opened and to his surprise, Lady McKensie strode into the office.

"Forgive me, but the student, Father Hardwicke. Where is the student who assisted Simon during the experiment?" she blurted.

"Haggett?"

"Is that his name?"

"Aye, Oswold Haggett."

"I must speak to him, Father," she said, her tone urgent.

"He was with MaryPryde the night she died. He may have seen something. Is he on duty? And what about Sister Rosamond? Did anyone ask if she saw anything?"

"Sister Rosamond has already said she saw nothing out of the ordinary." Father Hardwicke looked to the registrar. "Is Haggett on duty?"

The registrar shrugged his shoulders. "I've nae seen 'im since the guards took McKensie away."

Father Hardwicke furrowed his brow. "Is he down in the student dormitory?"

"Would ye 'ave me look?"

"If you would, please."

The registrar left the office with all the fresh authority he could impart. An orderly passed the doorway carrying a stack of blankets. "Move!" the registrar cried, pushing the orderly aside. The blankets fell to the floorboards as the registrar bustled down the hallway.

"I very much doubt he will be there," said Catherine, watching the irritated orderly gather the quilts back up. "Where is his home?"

Father Hardwicke rose and walked several paces to a cabinet. He pulled a thick ledger from a shelf, and then leafed through its yellowing pages. "Haggett. Stockton Heath." He looked up. "'Tis a five hour ride. Do you know of it?"

"I do. The village is on the road to my own home in Wells," she said, pulling on her riding gloves.

"I was just writing my defense for Charles, but if you can wait, I will accompany you if Haggett is not found in the dormitories."

"You are very kind, but I know the way quite well." She faced the priest. "I think it most important that you remain here with Charles, as your testimony will be invaluable tomorrow." Catherine walked to the doorway and waited for the registrar to confirm what she already knew to be true. She turned back with a catch in her voice. "I cannot thank you enough, Father."

Father Hardwicke rose from his chair and met her at the doorway. Taking her hands into his own, he could hear the heartfelt emotion in her voice. For the first time in his life, the priest was at a loss for words. He grasped her by the hands. "Though I cannot say what will happen, I do have faith, my dear." He closed his eyes. "That your faith might not rest in the wisdom of men, but in the power of God, for nothing is impossible with God..." His prayer was interrupted by the sound of heavy footsteps hurrying down the hallway. He opened his eyes to the sight of the registrar limping back.

"Hasn't been seen these three days," he wheezed, leaning against the wall to catch his breath.

Father Hardwicke turned to Catherine and raised his hand in the sign of the cross. "Go with God."

CHAPTER FORTY-THREE

"THE CUSTOM OF SINNING TAKES AWAY THE SENSE OF IT, THE
COURSE OF THE WORLD TAKES AWAY THE SHAME OF IT"
~ JOHN OWEN, 1642

Malmesbury House
Thursday, 10 March 1667
4:46 pm

amn the bitch! King Charles II sat alone, brooding before the fire in heavy contemplations. By turns both melancholy and consumed with a seething fury, he sat in his thick, velvet dressing gown and stared at the flames in the modest country house far from London. Privately mocked by his courtiers for its humble size, Malmesbury House was a favored retreat of the king. Once a safe refuge from the plague-ravaged city, and now, a place of solace from the sting of Barbara's temper, the country house was a place where he could retreat from his world and think. And think, he must, for the pretty, witty, and very young Nell Gwyn had stolen his heart. But, he loved his bewitching, tempestuous Barbara. And, he was married to the Spanish princess. He lifted a snifter from an Elizabethan side table and inhaled its thick, oaken aroma. He took another sip of the Augier Congiack, luxuriating in the 17th century French eau-de-vie, as the fiery amber liquid seared his royal throat, then fell back to his sorrowful ruminations.

His wife was largely insignificant. Fair of face she was not, and well she knew. Swaddled by the comforting rituals of her religion, she asked nothing more of him save permission to practice her cherished Catholic faith. And children. She desperately wished for children. *Alas, she was barren.* He had given her all the rope she desired to live the prayerful life she wished. And that was enough for her. As far as the queen was concerned, he was free to chase any fleeting fancy that caught his royal eye. Just as he had to her, she had given to him in his merry pursuit of feminine flesh, rope enough. *Rope enough to hang himself.*

He set the snifter back on the carved side table and fingered the two parchment letters that had been delivered that day by messenger. He did not recognize the dark green wax seal on the one letter, but they both carried the fragrance of his tempestuous, infuriating, beloved mistress. He held the letters to his nose and inhaled. He knew that spicy, citrus fragrance well, for he himself had created the perfume especially for Barbara. He turned the letter over. Fine, silken threads imbedded in the red wax dangled from the parchment. Though he was wont to do it, he pulled slowly at the thread until, at last, it sliced, razor-sharp, through the wax. He did not want to read the missive. He, in fact, dreaded her words. He had once, while she was heavy with his first child, had an *affaire du couer* with a nimble, buxom courtesan. Incensed in the extreme, Barbara threatened to kill the child at birth unless he dropped to his knees and begged her forgiveness before his entire court. *How she had humiliated him.* Yet, he begged her forgiveness willingly. He could not break the bond; so utterly bewitched was he by his sultry mistress. A dalliance with Nell would bring yet another swift and vicious retribution, of that he was sure, but this time he would not crawl back. He would not humiliate himself again, no matter her terms. *Nae, he would not.* He exhaled. *But he loved her.* He turned back to the flames that licked the stone hearth, his mind in sheer torment. *How could he possibly live without her?* He unfolded both letters, glancing at them with a wary eye.

A ferocious pounding on the front door's brass plate abruptly shattered his woeful lamentations. Seconds later, he heard riotous shouts ringing through the entry hall. He turned his head in time to see Wilmot, Killigrew and May burst into the chamber, laughing giddily, champagne bottles raised high over their bewigged heads.

"We've come to play!" cried Wilmot, skipping happily across the limestone floor.

"And play, we shall! Horse races on the lawn!" shouted Killegrew.

May dangled his bottle of champagne above the king's head. "And to the victor, goes the spoils…" he drawled, pointing to the entry hall behind them. The king turned around to see the luminous Nell Gwyn standing still in the doorway. She wore a tempting, low-cut gown of golden silks, backlit by the fading light of a late afternoon sun.

The king half-rose from his chair, stunned to silence by the young beauty. He saw the letters on the table. *Barbara.* He looked once more to Nell. She turned to walk away, then glanced back over her shoulder, her eyes taunting him to follow. Excited beyond all reason, King Charles II bent down and took the letters in hand as if to restrain himself. At the entrance, Nell bent down to straighten her skirts. She lifted her eyes, then took hold of the neckline of her gown and slowly pulled down, exposing her bare breasts for all to see. In the shocked silence, a single strawberry dropped from her cleavage. It hit the floor with a soft thud and bounced, rolling to a stop by her foot.

"Oops," she giggled, then pretty, witty Nell walked out the door with an unrepentant wink, to the raucous cheers of the three merry courtiers. The king flung the letters straight into the flames.

CHAPTER FORTY-FOUR

Stockton Heath
Buckinghamshire, England
Thursday, 10 March 1667
9:31 pm

Expert horsewoman that she was, even Catherine would admit to exhaustion as she at last approached the small village of Stockton Heath. Though the cold night air chilled her to the bone, she was grateful, for the chill kept her awake in the saddle. She had never been so tired in her life. As she drew closer to the village, she could see a lamplighter striking a flint to a lantern at the edge of town. Suddenly wide-awake, Catherine kicked Ganymeade and galloped toward the man.

"Excuse me, sir," she called out, drawing closer.

The man looked up in surprise at the sight of a lone woman riding in the night. "Aye. Can I 'elp ye, Miss?"

"Oswold Haggett, I'm looking for a man called Oswold Haggett. Do you know of him?"

"Aye, I do. He'd be the son o' Josiah Haggett." He pointed to a humble, thatched dwelling back down the road from whence she'd come. A single, golden light shone through a window. "Just there. Would ye like me t' lead th' way?"

"You are very kind, but I believe I can find it." Catherine turned her horse. "Thank you, sir," she called out, as she galloped back down the road, leaving the lamplighter staring in her wake.

Her nerves got the better of her as she stood before the stone cottage. Catherine stepped back from the low, blue door and collected herself. The sudden thought of Simon alone in the prison cell steeled her determination. She approached the door once more and banged on the planks. After a moment, the door opened. A weather-beaten old man gazed at her with an expectant curiosity. "Aye? Canna' help ye?"

"I…I am looking for Oswold Haggett. Is he here?"

Before Josiah could speak, Catherine felt a sharp pain knifing through her left side. She gasped and clutched at her abdomen. Josiah's eyes widened as he grabbed her by the waist to keep her from sagging to the ground. "Aye, Miss!" he cried out, at a complete loss for words with the unexpected night visitor.

The pain subsiding, Catherine eased herself down to a bench by the door. Josiah moved a pair of muddy work boots aside, then sat next to her. "Are ye all right, Miss?"

Catherine took a deep breath. "I will be." She turned to him with a wan smile. "I've just ridden from London and I'm afraid the long ride has gotten the better of me."

Josiah gave a low whistle. "From London? Just now?" He shook his head. "Aye, lass." He took in her fine woolen cloak and costly leather riding gloves. She was no miscreant. "I think ye'd best come inside an' rest a bit. When was th' last time ye ate?" he asked, helping her up. She did not resist his strong grip.

"This afternoon," she said, embarrassed to admit she had gone off with nothing but the packet Gussie had prepared in a rush.

"Why, tha's hours ago," he said, as he led her into the small, but inviting cottage. He pointed to a rocking chair before a well-tended fire in the keeping room. "Sit. Warm yer'self." Josiah went to a shelf mounted above a cooking grate and pulled down a loaf of bread and a half-wheel of cheddar cheese. Staring at the cheese, he scratched his head a moment, perplexed. "I 'ad a full wheel," he mumbled, then shook his head and reached for a wooden plate. He cut a generous chunk of the bread and cheese and set the plate in her lap. "Porridge won't take but a minute."

"Please do not go to any trouble," said Catherine.

"'Tis' no trouble, Miss." He jostled the coals to life, and then measured the oats and water into a sturdy pot on the grate. "Ye asked about my son. He's nae here, but can ye tell me why ye ask?"

Catherine hesitated, thinking to keep Simon's troubles to herself until she spoke to Oswold, but the man had a kind face and seemed genuinely concerned. Before she could speak, the latch on the front door rattled. Josiah turned from the cook pot as the door was thrown wide.

Oswold stood in the doorway, straw sprouting at odd angles from his hair and tunics. He looked to Catherine. "I saw you from the barn, Lady McKensie, an' I know why you're here." He saw his father's shocked expression and could not hold back the tears. "I'm so sorry, Da," he sobbed.

⚭

Oswold and Catherine sat warming themselves by the fire, as Josiah ladled from the iron pot. He handed them each a thirken of porridge and then eased himself down to the hearth, watching them eat. He could hardly believe Oswold's tale. "Two days, lad? Ye've been hiding in the barn fer two days? Whatever for?"

"I..I canna' say," whispered Oswold, staring at the floorboards.

Josiah set his hands to his knees, giving Oswold's response the full weight of his considerations. After a moment, he shook his head. "Nae. Tha' won't do." He leaned toward his son. "I 'spect ye'd best tell me the whole of it."

Oswold exhaled. *There is no escape.* Josiah fell silent as Oswold began to describe the experiment, speaking in great detail of MaryPryde, the blood transfusion, the sheep, and her sad fate.

At the mention of MaryPryde, Catherine could hold back no more. "Oswold, Simon has been arrested for murder!" she cried out, interrupting his story. "He has been in prison since MaryPryde's death. His trial is tomorrow. I must know—were you there?" she asked, her tone urgent. "Did you see anything?"

299

Oswold was clearly terrified. "I…I fear cannot speak to it, Milady."

Catherine's heart stopped, remembering Charles's words. *They will hang him, Catherine.*

A troubled Josiah spoke up. "Oswold, if you were a party to any of this, you must confess." He looked directly at Oswold. "Did you…hurt the girl?"

Oswold looked as though he had been struck. "No, Da!" cried Oswold, tears spilling down his cheeks. "I'd nae do such a terrible thing!"

"Did you speak to anyone? Did anyone else come into the room?" asked Catherine, desperate for any grain of hope.

Oswold looked miserable. "Aye," he whispered.

Catherine leaned forward, tense in anticipation. "Who?" she exclaimed. "Who else was there?"

Oswold closed his eyes, reliving the horrible moments. He looked as though he would be sick. Tears spilled once more.

"Palgrave," he sobbed. "Palgrave was there!"

"Dr. Palgrave?! What was he doing in the room?" she asked in confusion.

Oswold fell into an agonizing silence.

"Oswold," said Josiah in a tone that brooked no nonsense. "Compose yer'self, an' answer Lady McKensie."

Oswold choked back the tears. "He said 'e would dismiss me from medical school if I spoke of it." He turned to Catherine. "Milady, my father will lose the farm if I'm sent down. He will lose everything!"

Josiah clasped a firm hand on Oswold's back. "Leave the worryin' t' me, son. Tell Lady McKensie what she needs to know. Now."

A violent mix of anger and relief spilled over as, at last, Oswold jumped from the chair and set free the secret that had tormented him for days. "'E killed her!" he cried, pacing before the fire.

Catherine looked up, sharply. "What? He did what?"

Oswold began to sob once more. "'E…'e took a pillow an' 'eld it over her face. She was shakin' and thrashin' an' 'e said it were the devil, so's 'e killed MaryPryde before me own eyes." Oswold fell to his knees, grasping her by the hands. Oh, it were an awful thing to see, Lady McKensie. It were just awful." He began to shake at the memory.

"God's heart," whispered Josiah. He rose and walked slowly back to the shelf, trying to absorb the enormity of what his son had witnessed. He reached behind a pot and retrieved a jug. He pulled the cork, and handed it to Oswold. "'Ere, son. Take a wallop."

"He is innocent," Catherine whispered, as though not quite understanding what she had just heard. "Innocent!" she cried, jumping from the chair. "We've got to go back to London! We have to leave—we have to leave now!" Another cramp ripped through her abdomen. She buckled at the knees, and then fell to the hearth grasping her stomach.

"Lady McKensie!" shouted Oswold. "What is it? What is wrong?"

Catherine tried to rise. "I must go back to London! Please bring my horse." She looked to Oswold, desperation mounting. "You must come with me and testify on Simon's behalf!" She closed her eyes and breathed heavily as another pain ripped at her side.

"Of course, Lady McKensie. Of course I will testify," said Oswold, deeply concerned. "But, I dinna' think ye should ride." He helped her to her feet, and then led her to the rope bed on the opposite side of the keeping room.

"Have ye had these pains before, Milady?" whispered Oswold, as he settled her on the bed.

She looked at him with a mixture of alarm and sadness at the impossible predicament she was in. "Just today." She hesitated. "I am with child."

Oswold drew back. "Ye canna' go back to London, Milady!

Ye need t' rest. Ye may well lose the baby."

"If the baby is to be lost, I cannot stop it. But Simon needs help. He needs you to testify and I *will* be there."

"Dinna' worry, Milady." Relief washing over her, Catherine lay back on the bed for a moment, holding her side. Oswold rose to cover her with a quilt from a trunk at the foot of the bed. When he looked back, Catherine was fast asleep.

CHAPTER FORTY-FIVE

"I'M ABOUT TO TAKE MY LAST VOYAGE, A
GREAT LEAP INTO THE DARK."
~ THOMAS HOBBES

The Public Office
Bow Street Magistrate
London, England
Friday, 11 March 1667
9:42am

The mayor and Viola fought their way through the
frenzied crowds that had gathered outside the Public
Office. Men, women, even children pushed and shoved each
other toward the entrance, fighting to secure one of the fifty
coveted spaces in the standing gallery of the magnificent trial
hall. On the ground, torn and dirty Gazette handbills littered
the courthouse steps.

"Where on God's earth is Catherine?" asked Viola, fearing
for her niece. "Charles said she rode to Stockton Heath last
night," she said, shaking her head in disbelief. "I cannot
imagine what for?"

"She must have had her reasons, though I truly am at a loss
as to why she is not here," said Cecil, with only a slight touch of
reassurance. He looked about, greatly troubled, himself.

"What could have happened?" fretted Viola. "I am terribly
concerned."

"Catherine is an excellent horsewoman, sweetings. She will
be here," he said, more to convince himself.

"Oi! Look at th' grand lady!" cried a woman in rags, grabbing
at the silken fabric of Viola's gown. "Are ye the murderer's

mum?" she taunted, pointing at a handbill with the lurid story in the center column.

Viola slapped the woman. "Get away!" Cecil took Viola by the arm and pulled her through the throng. "Did you see that awful woman?" cried Viola. "The very idea, pulling at my sleeves with her filthy hands!" She set her handkerchief to her nose to avoid the overwhelming stench from the crowd as they shoved their way into the building.

Cecil led Viola into the courtroom. Forgetting for the moment the occasion that led them there, Viola, like all who saw the immense chamber for the first time, stared in open-mouthed astonishment at its hushed splendor. The walls of the room were lined to the ceiling with paned windows. At the far end, an immense stone fireplace warmed the chamber, and high above it all was a soaring, box-beamed ceiling, crafted with walnut-stained timbers. In the center of each boxed panel, a gold leaf star gleamed in the late morning light.

Set before the fireplace was a wide, carved table reserved for the magistrate. Off to the side of the magistrate's table, two rows of benches lined the wall beneath the windows for the jury, and in the formal gallery facing the judge were three more rows of benches, arranged much like the pews in church. Opposite the jury, the bespectacled man from the Gazette sat ready. Overcome by the gravity of the circumstances, Viola stopped short and reached for the mayor. "Oh, Cecil. This cannot be. It just cannot be." She sank to the bench in the second row before she swooned.

Ledger in hand, Charles walked in after them, followed by Robert Boyle, each taking a seat on the bench in the front row. Boyle, looking grim but resolute, opened his own ledger and began to review his notes. Father Hardwicke joined the apprehensive men on the bench as they waited their turn to testify. In the back, the unruly crowd who had pushed their way into the standing gallery fell to silence as five beautifully dressed women walked through the crowd to the third row, taking their seats on the bench.

"I canna' see, Mummy," said a small girl with a loud voice in the standing area. She jumped up and down, craning her neck to see over the benches. "Tha' lady's hat is too big."

Margaret Cavendish, in a very wide, black taffeta hat, turned slightly and gave a formal nod to the girl, though she did not remove her headpiece. Neither did Aphra Behn, Elizabeth Wilbraham, Bathusa Makin or Lady Phillipa Dillworth.

"Cooee, look at them fine ladies," whispered a little boy of about ten to his mother. The mother nodded, her mouth agape at the sight. "Oi, just look at 'em!" she said, impressed herself by the finery.

On the opposite side, Godfrey Palgrave sat alone. He had taken great pains to comb his hair and wore his cleanest tunic for the momentous occasion. He looked neither left nor right, but stared straight toward the magistrate's table as the jury filed in and took their seats on the side benches. Not a single soul sat with him.

Viola looked around the room, desperate to find Catherine, to no avail. The door behind the magistrate's table opened. The crowd fell silent once more as the bailiff led Simon to a stand between the table and the jury.

The sight of him was a shock to Viola, for he looked frightful. In just three days time, he seemed to have lost weight. His eyes were circled dark with exhaustion. His hair was matted. His torn, filthy tunics hung loose and hindered his path as he tried to balance in the irons that shackled his feet. Viola involuntarily cried out. "Simon!"

Simon looked up at the sound of his name, and saw the crowd of friends that had formed in his defense. At the back of the chamber, Gussie and Archie had joined the crowd in the standing gallery. Gussie, in a flowered cap, smiled and gave a small wave before Archie silenced her in deference to the solemn occasion. Simon nearly broke down at the loyalty. He craned his neck, searching for Catherine. *Where is she?* He looked back to Viola, a troubled, questioning look upon his face. In anguish, Viola shook her head. *No.*

∽∾

"Order!!" shouted the bailiff. Simon felt the pit of his stomach drop. Though he refused to think upon the worst, he began to tremble with dread. *He had lost her. She was too ashamed to come.* He could barely breathe. The door opened once more. A hush fell over the crowd as the judge, dressed in formal black robes, walked into the chamber and took his chair. He took a moment to read through the indictments set before him, and then the magistrate lifted his head and looked over to Simon at the stand. Simon, staring down to the scarred, wooden floor, felt every single pair of eyes upon him.

"We assemble here this day at the behest of the accuser, Doctor Godfrey Palgrave," the judge began. "The defendant, the physick Simon McKensie, of St. Bartholomew's Hospital, is accused of two concurrent charges. The first: a charge of grave robbing, exhumation and the illegal dissection and dismemberment of the mendicant order."

A wild roar went up through the chamber. Simon watched as Viola, horrified by the jeers and crude shouts from the standing gallery, buried her face in Cecil's cloak. *How could he face her — how could he face any of them, again?* The bailiff held his hand high. "Order!" he bellowed. "Order!" He kept his hand raised until quiet was restored.

The judge turned to Simon. "How do you plead to the first charge?"

Despite his fear, Simon lifted his chin and spoke loudly and clearly. "Not guilty."

"Grave-robbin' thief!" shouted a man at the front of the gallery.

"'Tis' a sin against God, 'imself" shouted another. The crowd shouted its approval of that righteous assessment.

"Order!" cried the bailiff once more.

The judge waited until the crowd settled. "As to the second charge of the murder of Miss MaryPryde Beckwith." he continued. "How do you plead?"

"Not guilty, your honor!"

The gallery erupted.

"Hang 'em!" the crowd shouted, now thirsting for blood. "Hang 'im by th' neck 'til 'e's dead!"

Simon ducked as a man threw a half-eaten apple at him, missing his head by inches. It banged off the stand and landed on the magistrate's table, rolling to a stop on his papers. A guard in the standing gallery grabbed the man and to the outraged cries of the crowd, hauled him from the courtroom. Another man shoved his way in to take his place.

"I'll not tolerate this behavior," shouted the judge, banging on the table with his hand, "or I shall clear the courtroom!" He caught the eye of the bailiff and waved toward the apple. "Remove this."

"Order!" shouted the bailiff. "Fer the last time, ORDER!"

"Who here stands to this man's defense?" called out the magistrate, as the crowd settled once again.

Simon exhaled in relief as he watched Father Hardwicke rise. "I do." The boisterous gallery fell to silence in deference to a man of the cloth in their midst.

"Please come forward."

Father Hardwicke made his way to the front, giving an encouraging nod to Simon as he stepped to the witness stand. He took a deep breath, and then turned to the jury. "I am Father Thomas Hardwicke, Head Administrator of St. Bartholomew's-The-Less Hospital. I have known the defendant for over six years. In that time, I have watched this young man rise from earnest scholar to caring resident, to licensed physick. He is, by many times over, the most intelligent of men, and a dedicated man of science. In his endless pursuit of knowledge, he hath turned the full breadth of his intelligence to discovery in ways that will advance scientific knowledge for the betterment of us all."

Humbled by the praise, Simon's eyes glistened as Father Hardwicke spoke.

"I, and I alone, sanctioned the experiment at St. Bartholomew's, just as I sanctioned the dissection of the human body after a death for the knowledge gained," said Father Hardwicke. "And as to the experiment, the patient was duly informed several times over to the dangers of such a course, and yet, she gave her full consent to the process, because she wished to be a part of scientific discovery—and in that endeavor, she has been. We must be grateful to both MaryPryde Beckwith and Simon McKensie for advancing scientific knowledge one more increment. Not only do I well and truly believe this man to be innocent of the dissections for the betterment of us all, I proclaim Simon McKensie innocent of the charge of murder!"

"Here, here!" shouted the fickle crowd, easily swayed by a well-versed argument. "Here, here!"

Simon managed a half-smile to Father Hardwicke as the priest returned to his place on the bench to confer with Cecil and Charles.

"Is there anyone else who wishes to testify on this defendant's behalf?"

"I do," called out Robert Boyle.

"Come forward."

As the scientist made his way to the witness stand, Simon searched the courtroom once more, in vain hopes that Catherine had slipped into the crowd. Disconsolate by her absence, he turned his attention to the older man, nodding his gratitude to Boyle as he passed to take the stand.

Boyle waited for the full attention of the noisy gallery. "I am Robert Boyle, chymist of Oxford University, scientific advisor to King Charles II, and humble servant of God," he shouted. The crowd fell to a respectful silence at the mention of

Oxford, the King and God, himself. "I stand before you today in defense of a fellow scientist." He gazed upon the assembly for a moment, and then continued, raising his voice for all to hear. "The book of nature is a fine and large piece of tapestry rolled up," he shouted, "which we are not able to see all at once, but must be content to wait for the discovery of it's beauty and symmetry, little by little, as it gradually comes to be more and more unfolded."

The standing crowd looked to one another, baffled in their limited imaginings, in an attempt to make sense of his words. Simon glanced to the jury, praying they would understand Boyle's intellectual ways.

"The experiments of Simon McKensie are but one more piece of that fine and large tapestry that has begun to unfold before us in our quest to understand nature and the human body and even when we find not what we seek, we find something as well worth seeking as what we missed."

In the gallery, several men cleared their throats and a baby, grasped tight in her mother's arms, began to fuss. To Simon's dismay, the crowd at the back was growing bored with the scientists' high-minded testimony.

Ignoring the restless rasps, Boyle continued. "In our efforts to understand the human body, these experiments become invaluable. As a physick, Simon McKensie was responsible for saving the lives of many when the plague struck the village of Wells. That research may be unknown to most, but his efforts were notable in the extreme for those of us who attempt daily to understand disease and its spread. Were it not for Doctor McKensie and his research on the practice of isolation, most in Wells would have perished."

Simon looked at the jury once more. To a man they were attentive, leaning forward to hear each word. His spirits lifted slightly.

"We must ask ourselves if we prefer to live in the darkness of our ignorance, or in the infinite light of scientific knowledge? I think it far preferable to live in the light of knowledge, for God would not have made the universe as it is unless He intends us to understand it."

As the audience weighed those words, Boyle stepped down and took his seat on the bench to confer with Charles and the mayor. Someone from the back of the room began to clap. Another man clapped, then the full balance of the crowd stepped forward and applauded.

"Order," shouted the bailiff, though with a softer tone. "Order!" he called out until the gallery quieted down.

"Is there anyone else who will stand to the defendants innocence?" asked the magistrate.

None stood. "Then we shall hear from the accuser. Will Doctor Palgrave come forward?"

"Aye, I will." Palgrave walked to the stand and took his place, not deigning to look at Simon. "I am Doctor Godfrey Palgrave, surgeon at St. Bartholomew's. I stand today against the actions taken by this man," he stated, his voice loud and sure. Palgrave walked to the magistrate's table and held up one of the dissection drawings, painstaking in its bloody detail. "This drawing is but one of hundreds," he said, as he paraded the parchment before the jury."

Simon's heart dropped once more as several members of the jury looked away, revolted by the sight.

"Look at it!" Palgrave screeched to the jury. Still more turned away. "This man paid *thieves* to exhume those who could not speak for themselves. He ripped from the ground those whom God had taken into his merciful arms." Palgrave's voice dropped to a dramatic tone. "He butchered these defenseless souls for whom no one cared." Palgrave waved the parchment once more. "T'was a lawless act, no matter the scientific benefit. Illegal in the extreme. Punishable by *death*. You have but to ask the defendant who stands before you this day. Did he commit these exhumation crimes? The initials on each and every illustration attest in full to that." He turned to Simon, jabbing his finger toward the signature. "Is this your mark? Before God and these witnesses, will you stand here today and deny that you are the architect of these blasphemous acts?"

Simon lifted his chin. "I'll not deny it." The crowd, as one, gasped at the drama unfolding before them. "The scientific research is mine and mine alone."

The crowd, emotions high and turning on a penny, began to hiss at Simon. The hisses turned to outright condemnation as the full weight of his confession took hold. Palgrave returned to the stand and waited until the gallery quieted down.

"And then...poor, lamentable MaryPryde Beckwith. An innocent, young woman coerced by the defendant into a godless experiment. The victim of a blood transfusion – from no less than a common farm animal! The whole of life laid before her, this beautiful young woman of but seventeen years nae lies dead by the direct hand of this man!" he shouted, pointing to Simon.

The crowd cried out a violent condemnation of the murder. Simon could barely breathe, such was the profound sorrow and fear that fell like a mantle around his soul.

"She trusted this man and by his hand, and his hand alone, she this day lies dead in the ground!" Palgrave screamed, his face turning purple with a fervid wrath. "He hath performed these acts. He hath confessed to these acts. Find him guilty!!"

"Hang 'im!" shouted voices from crowd once more. "Hang 'im by the neck!"

Palgrave turned to Simon with a twisted sneer, then, to the raucous cries of the gallery, walked back to his place on the bench.

The magistrate waited until the bailiff silenced the crowd. Simon began to shake in the crowded, foul-smelling courtroom, for he knew what lay ahead.

"Are there any other accusers?" asked the judge.

Viola clutched the arms of both Cecil and Charles. She turned her head toward the back of the room, looking in vain for Catherine. She began to cry from the anguish.

None stood. "Very well," intoned the judge. He turned to the jury. "Gentlemen, it is your sworn duty to confer between yourselves and decide this defendants guilt or innocence. Please gather by the fire, discuss the facts of the case, and come to a decision."

As one, the jury stood and walked to the back of the room. Simon watched as nearly everyone assembled in the chamber leaned forward in an attempt to catch a word or two, to no avail. The theater of it all was too much for one woman in the standing gallery who fainted and had to be carried from the chamber. Simon, himself, could hear nothing save the deafening sound of his own pounding heart.

At length, the jury walked back to the benches. Simon searched every face for some betrayal of the verdict, but none dared glance his way. He inhaled deeply, in an attempt to keep from passing out. He thought his knees would buckle for the fear. He grasped the stand, searching once more for Catherine, with the knowledge that if the verdict were guilty, they would walk him straight to the gallows. *He may never see her again.*

The magistrate addressed the jury. "Have you reached a verdict?"

A well-dressed gentleman at the end of the front bench nodded. "Aye, we have, sir."

The man from the Gazette took his quill in hand, dipped its point into an inkpot, and readied himself to transcribe what was to come next.

"Will the jury please rise?"

Simon held his breath as all members of the jury stood. None looked toward him. The room began to spin.

"To the first charge of grave-robbing, exhumation, dissection and dismemberment of the mendicant order, what say you?"

As one, the jury spoke. "Guilty as charged, sir."

Viola cried out, grasping at Charles and Cecil.

"To the second charge of the murder of MaryPryde Beckwith, what say you?"

The jury spoke once more. "Guilty as charged, sir."

Viola fainted. The crowd, as one, thundered their approval at the verdicts. A brawl commenced in the gallery between two men fighting for a better view.

"Guards!" shouted the magistrate. "Remove the prisoner while I deliberate punishment."

Pandemonium raged in the courtroom as the guards took Simon by the arms and pulled him, stumbling, through the door at the back of the chamber. Unheard over the shouts, cheers and the fisticuffs, the door at the front was thrown wide. Catherine, Oswold and Josiah burst into the room, shoving their way through the gallery toward the magistrate's table.

"Catherine!" Viola rushed to gather her niece into her arms. "I was so worried!" she cried.

Catherine pulled from her aunt's grasp. "Arrest him!" shouted Catherine, pointing at Palgrave.

The onlookers, sensing more drama, stood where they were, staring at Catherine. They fell silent.

Catherine pulled Oswold to the magistrate's table. "This man saw it all," she shouted once more. "Arrest Dr. Palgrave for the murder of MaryPryde Beckwith!"

The judge looked to Oswold. "Is this true? Were you a witness to the death of Miss Beckwith?"

A trembling Oswold looked as though he were about to faint. "I was, sir." He dared a glance to an enraged Palgrave. "I...I saw everything."

"Return the defendant to the stand," ordered the magistrate.

"Damn you, Haggett!" shouted Palgrave as he jumped from the bench and began to shove his way toward the door. Two burly men in the gallery grabbed him as he passed. Hauling him unceremoniously back into the courtroom, they handed him over to the guards who shackled him to prevent a further attempt at flight.

As the guards escorted Simon back to the magistrate, he stopped short, his heart soaring at the sight of Catherine at the judge's table. Relief flooded over him. "Catherine," he breathed. Were it not for the irons that bound his feet, nothing could have kept him from her.

The magistrate looked at Oswold. "What say you?" he commanded.

Palgrave raged against the irons that bound him. "Damn you forever to hell!" he shouted, spitting at Oswold. "Depart from me, you cursed, into the eternal fire prepared for the devil!!"

Oswold recoiled from the unbalanced physick. Josiah, standing calmly by, nodded to his son. "Go on, boyo. He canna' hurt you, nae."

Oswold took a deep breath, relieved to unburden his soul. "'e did it!" he cried, pointing at Palgrave. "That night, after th' experiment, Doctor Palgrave came inta' the room shouting terrible curses at Miss Beckwith, scarin' 'er so's that she started shakin.' 'E were frightened by the sight of her, so's 'e shouted more. She couldn'a stop shakin, so's 'e took a pillow and held it over her face. Oh, it were an awful sight, sir. She couldn'a breathe. I begged 'im to let go. I tried to pull him away, but he just stood over her, holdin' th' pillow until she didna' move anymore." Oswold began to cry. "It weren't Dr. McKensie at all, and it weren't the experiment." The cries became sobs. "It were Doctor Palgrave who did it—he killed her, 'e did, an' I saw 'im do it!" Oswold leaned on the table, his tears spilling onto the parchments. "Ah, MaryPryde," he whispered. "I saw 'im do it," he sobbed softly.

The crowd was transfixed. "I believe the lad," shouted one man. "Me, too," shouted another. Within moments, the sentiment had swung back to Simon. "Arrest the bastard!" cried one more.

The magistrate raised his hand to silence the crowd. He looked to the bailiff and nodded.

"Order!" shouted the bailiff. "Order!" The gallery fell quiet.

"Doctor Godfrey Palgrave, you have been accused of the murder of Miss MaryPryde Beckwith."

"No!" shouted Palgrave, straining against the irons. "Tis' an abominable lie!"

"I hereby remand you to Clink Prison to await trial to commence in one weeks time," pronounced the judge.

The gallery cried out once more. "Murderer!" they shouted as one.

The judge looked to Simon, standing silent before him. "Based on the testimony given by this man, I hereby abrogate you of the charge of murder."

Against the raucous cheers of the gallery, the judge looked once more to the bailiff to silence the crowd.

"Order! ORDER!"

The judge continued in the now silent chamber. "However, as to the first allegation, you have been found…guilty as charged."

The blood drained from Simon's face. In a haze, he looked to Catherine, searching for her forgiveness. She clung to Charles and Viola in tears. Catherine turned toward the back of the room as though looking for a miracle.

The judge took a moment. "Simon McKensie, on this eleventh day of March, in the year of our Lord, one thousand six hundred sixty seven, you are hereby sentenced to death."

"No!" cried Catherine, bending over, clutching her stomach in anguish.

"Guards, escort the prisoner to the gallows."

Catherine watched as the guards took hold of Simon and dragged him from chamber. She pulled from Viola's grasp and ran toward him, but the gallery, bursting through the doorway to race to the prison yard, pushed her back. "Simon," she cried, glimpsing the top of his head above the crowd of people now choking the lane outside.

"Catherine!" Simon shouted back, straining from the guards, trying to reach for her. "I'm...I'm sorry."

Catherine shoved her way to the street where a riotous crowd had formed behind the prisoner. A hanging was exactly what they had come for and by all means, they were prepared to make a day of it. Wicker baskets and blankets were produced. Men on horseback rode up and down the lane shouting out the verdict, adding to the chaos. Cheers and excitable cries drew more people into the throng as the procession swelled into the hundreds. Small children skipped happily toward the prison courtyard, in giddy anticipation of the sweet treats hidden deep in their mother's pockets for the half-hour walk to the Clink.

<hr />

Mr. Fitch steered the excitable horses through the procession, shouting warnings to the people in his path. Inside, a tearful Viola, Charles and Cecil searched through the side windows for Catherine. Gussie and Archie looked through the rear. "Tis a true horror, Cecil," cried Viola. "Is there nothing that can be done?"

"I fear nothing save a miracle will help the lad," whispered Cecil.

"Charles? Is there no one? Perhaps at the Inns of Court?"

"I'm afraid not, Aunt Viola. Once the judge has rendered his verdict, the punishment is swift...and final."

CHAPTER FORTY-SIX

Clink Prison
Southwark, London
Friday, 11 March 1667
12:34 pm

The groundswell could be heard for nearly a mile. At first a low rumble, then the bedlam grew to an ungodly roar as a multitude of heads became visible over the rise toward Clink. Men charged toward the prison on horseback, fighting to secure a place in the courtyard for their families at the front of the low barricade set before the hanging platform. One boy of about twelve stood with his hands on the wooden rail staring up at the thick, twisted rope, transfixed. Despite the raucous laughs and merriment that surrounded him, he could not take his eyes from the noose that swung gently in the breeze. He shuddered.

"There he is!" cried the boy's father, pointing toward the lane where the guards were pulling Simon toward the platform. The crowd rushed the barricade.

Catherine, catching up to Simon and the guards, ran to stand in front of them, blocking their path to the gallows steps.

"Step aside, Miss," ordered one of the guards.

"Catherine!" cried Simon, trying to pull from their grasp. The guards jerked him back.

"I am Lady McKensie," she said, forcefully, "and I will not move. I must be allowed to speak to my husband." She stood her ground in defiance, daring to challenge the guards nearly twice her size.

The guards looked to one another, then nodded, stepping slightly aside. They did not, however, let go.

Catherine ran to Simon and held him as best as she could,

grateful to be with him once more. "I have tried everything I could think of, Simon. I…I do not know what else to do," she faltered. She clung to him, unable to speak in her profound sorrow.

"There is nothing else to be done. I knew this day could come, and yet, in my arrogance, I honestly did not think it would. You will never know how sorry I am to have brought you into my troubles," he said, choking back tears. "I should never have asked you to be my wife." He could barely breathe. Terror clung to him as much as the sadness. "I…I am afraid, Catherine."

"I would not trade one single day of my life with you," she said, through her own tears. "I love you with all my heart."

Fitch pulled the carriage up next to the prison. The family made their way through the crowd toward Catherine and Simon. The costly clothing they wore caused the crowd to move back in awe as they passed. Viola looked dazed as the women in the crowd reached out to grab at the lace on her gown. This time, she felt none of it.

"Tha's it," growled the guard. He pulled Simon from Catherine's grasp and turned him toward the platform beneath the rope.

Catherine clung to Charles as Simon faced the steps. One by one, Simon climbed the treads, his heart pounding, his knees shaking, each step closer toward the unthinkable. He reached the scaffold. The noose dangled before him. He closed his eyes and inhaled. He felt the fresh breeze across his face, ruffling his hair. When he opened his eyes, Father Hardwicke stood before him, bible in hand. The magistrate stood behind him. The priest looked to Simon, deeply troubled, his eyes glistening. He had no words. Simon simply nodded. "Aye." Father Hardwicke watched in disbelief as the rope was lowered.

The guard reached up and pulled it around Simon's head. Simon could feel the weight of the rope sitting solidly around his neck. The course fibers scratched his skin. He began to tremble.

The crowd, falling silent in anticipation of the imminent hanging, lowered their heads in reverence. The rope tightened. Father Hardwicke raised his voice. "Almighty God," he shouted, "look upon this your servant, lying in great weakness, and comfort him with the promise of life everlasting."

Simon felt the rope pull against his neck. He closed his eyes. A strange peace fell over him.

"Have mercy on your serv—"

In the distance, an unholy commotion interrupted the priest. The startled crowd looked back to see a horse and rider galloping furiously toward the prison yard.

"Stop!" the rider shouted, dust billowing in his wake. "Stop!" he cried out once more, pulling the horse up short at the barricade. The crowd fell silent at the majesty of his royal attire.

Simon opened his eyes. He stared at the rider in disbelief, unsure if the moment was real or a cunning trick of the mind.

Tobias Stokes mounted the platform and produced a parchment scroll. "You are the physick, Simon McKensie, are you not?"

"Yes," whispered Simon, utterly confounded.

Tobias faced the crowd. He handed the parchment to the magistrate.

"Hang 'im!" shouted a man at the front.

"Silence!" The judge unrolled the scroll. After a moment, he stepped to the edge of the platform. He raised his voice and read from the parchment. "The King's most Excellent Majesty, taking into his gracious and serious consideration the practical contributions brought forth by the scientific experiments of this prisoner, except and always foreprized out of a free and general pardon, hath this day granted full pardon to this prisoner." The magistrate turned to Simon and handed him the scroll. "By order of King Charles II, Simon McKensie you are a free man."

CHAPTER FORTY-SEVEN

"LOVE WILL FIND A WAY"
~ PROVERBS

St. Bartholomew's Hospital
Friday, 25 March 1667
8:54 pm

"Nae, sir. I would prefer t' wait fer another doctor, if ye don't mind," whispered a woman at the registrar's desk, glancing sidelong at Simon. Blood dripped down her cheek from a wicked gash across her forehead. Holding a tattered cloth to her wound, she leaned closer the registrar. "Ain't 'e McKensie? Ain't 'e th' physick what pulled them dead bodies from th' ground?" She shuddered. "Oooh, an' I couldn'a bear 'im touchin' me fer the thought of it!"

Simon sighed. She was the ninth patient that day that had seen the Gazette handbills or heard the gossip that had been swirling around the West End since the trial two weeks before.

"'E's th' only physick available at the moment, so's it's 'im or it's no one," groused the overworked registrar, toting up his ledgers.

The woman backed toward the doorway, holding the blood-soaked cloth to her head. "No one, then. I'll nae have tha' ghoul stitchin' up m'e conk," she avowed. The door slamming on her way out echoed throughout the great hall.

The registrar cocked an eyebrow toward Simon. "Oi. Seems t' be a common enough sentiment these days," he taunted, with a disdainful shrug of the shoulders. Ignoring Simon, the registrar dipped his quill into an inkpot, shook off the excess, and returned to his inventory counts.

Simon turned from the peevish little man and walked toward

the now vacant dissection theater. It had been stripped of his desk, Catherine's illustration table, and the dissection platform. Even the student platform had been dismantled. The room had changed. In fact, in the two weeks since his trial, everything had changed. After a public trial, Godfrey Palgrave had been found guilty, sentenced to death, and hung from the gallows at Clink to the roaring cheers of a vengeful crowd. At Bealeton House, Viola and Cecil were making preparations to return to the abbey. Though she would not speak to it, Simon knew that Viola's invitations to the mid-winter celebrations at the height of London's social festivities had not come. *Nor would they.* They would never come, for Simon was now tainted. *The mere accusation of murder had been enough.* No matter that he was innocent of the charge, no matter that he had been pardoned by King Charles II, himself, Simon was tainted, and that taint had spread not only to the family, but it had spread to the hospital. The guilt was overwhelming. People avoided him on the street. Social calls had been tactfully cancelled. Even Robert Boyle had sent his regrets when Simon suggested a meeting. Though the words were kind, his note dripped with an unspoken fear that the poisonous taint would spread to Boyle, himself.

Father Hardwicke had called him into the offices. "The dissectory closure is not permanent, lad," said the priest, with a sympathetic pat on the shoulder. "But, I am afraid that any sort of controversy causes our benefactors to tighten the purse strings," he set both hands on the back of the chair and whispered into Simon's ear for emphasis, "and that outcome is to be avoided at all costs."

It was as though the great spool of his life had suddenly become unwound, and Simon did not know where or how to pick up the thread to begin again. What would he do without his research? His experiments? *His patients?* He leaned against the doorframe of the empty dissectory. A sad, desolation overwhelmed him as he began to comprehend the full extent of the accusations. The facts did not matter. People believed what they heard, and the gossip was rampant. Nothing he did made anything better. *Nothing would ever be the same.* The only constant in his life was Catherine. As he gazed into the vacant chamber, he knew for certain that she would forever be by his side. In the dim light of a single torch, he looked down to his pocket watch. His shift was over.

⚬∞⚬

The house was dark when a weary Simon climbed the steps to Bealeton House. He thought of hiring a hackney, but he preferred this night to walk. He needed to be alone with his thoughts. It was a clear, cool night, yet he could still smell the faint scent of smoke in the air. They had gotten used to the smoke, much as they had the vinegar. He barely noticed it now. He set his fingers on the latch, and then turned back and sat down wearily on the steps, trying to sort out what had become of his life. Behind him, the door opened.

"Simon."

Catherine stood in the doorway, holding her hand out to him. The worries that tied his stomach in knots through the day melted at the sight of her.

"Come inside," she said, her voice soft and warm.

Shedding his cloak, Simon followed her into the dining room where two plates of sliced lamb and boiled carrots sat under the glow of the candelabras. For some strange reason, the dull orange of the carrots lifted his gray spirits for a moment. Viola and Cecil had long since eaten and had retired for the night. Simon and Catherine were alone. Simon sank into the chair. He took the fork in hand, then set it down and shook his head. He had no appetite.

"I'm so very sorry, Catherine. I have caused irreparable harm to you and your family." He looked miserable.

Her smile was gentle. "We know the truth, Simon, and if we all agree, which we do, then no one else's opinions or actions can matter in the least."

"But your aunt, is she not distressed by the spurned invitations? Are you not troubled by the gossip? The condemnations?" He picked at the lamb. "Viola must be devastated."

"I believe that if this happened several years ago, she would have taken straight to her bed, but this day, she seems to have taken the rejection with a pinch of salt. She is a changed woman since she married the mayor. Much has happened to both soften and harden her to the whims of London society, and I can say with confidence that she is quite relieved to return to the abbey. With the mayor to take care of, she will find contentment in the country and I know the mayor feels the same."

Simon caught his reflection in the silver candlesticks. He tilted his head, considering the luxury of his surroundings, and then reached over to play his fingers across the fine, silver filigree. "I miss the cottage," he said, at length. He gestured to the expansive dining room. "I do not belong in such fashionable surroundings. And now, I do not belong at the hospital, either. In truth, I fear that I do not belong anywhere." He searched her eyes. "I honestly do not know what the future holds."

Since the trial, the wracking pains had eased with no issue, and Catherine had had plenty of time to think. She considered his words a moment, and then pulled a letter from her pocket. She glanced down to the careful penmanship. "This is a letter from Uncle George. In the colonies." She unfolded the wrinkled, well-worn parchment and spread the letter before Simon. He picked it up and held the letter to the candelabra, but the script was difficult to read in the pale light. He looked to her, questioning.

"Charles wrote to tell my uncle of our marriage and to reassure him that that we all had survived the fire. He sends his very best wishes…" she paused, not quite knowing how he would accept the next bit of news, "…and has extended an invitation."

Simon looked up in surprise. "An invitation? To what? The colonies?"

"He writes that your skills are much in demand in Boston, as the city is growing by the day." She reached for the letter. "It seems that physicks are desperately needed," she smiled.

It took a full minute for Simon to absorb her words. "You would consider sailing to the colonies? You would leave your aunt? Your brother?" Simon asked, incredulous. "You would leave England?"

"It was Aunt Viola's idea that we accept Uncle George's invitation."

"You've spoken to her about this?" he asked, astonished that she would even consider the proposal.

"I have spoken to both Aunt Viola and Charles. It is not out of the realm of possibilities that she would one day sail herself, once the mayor is completely well, as would Charles." Catherine smiled a mischievous smile. "My aunt is full of surprises." She looked down, modest in her admission. "It would seem I favor her in that regard."

Simon considered the tempting prospect. "What did Charles say? Do you think he would consider joining us?"

"Charles would like to finish his legal training at Lincoln's Inn, and intends to remain in London to manage both estates with help from our solicitor and the mayor. Although he wishes to remain in his current lodgings, he has plans to expand the resources of both Bealeton House and the Abbey. He will stay at the Inns of Court for the next three years of his training, and after that, I believe he would like to join the East India Company, in honor of Father."

"A fitting tribute, indeed." Simon looked dubious. "When would such a crossing take place? If Charles intends to remain in London, I suppose there would not be much to do but pack our trunks." He stared at her, a spark of excitement beginning to catch fire. "You would seriously consider such an undertaking, Catherine?"

"The *Recovery* sails in three weeks time."

They sat quiet at the table, considering the monumental decision they were about to make. The French porcelain clock on the sideboard chimed, breaking the silence. Simon took Catherine's hand into his own. "What is it you wish to do?" he asked, his voice soft with emotion. "

Catherine took a deep breath, anger flashing in her eyes. "They have dismantled your dissectory and put a stop to your experiments, and to be honest, Simon, it is clear to me that you are not content, nor will you ever be, in treating patients who do not trust you for wont of the libelous handbills from the London Gazette. It is an insult to a man of your ability and intellect, and I cannot think for one moment that you would wish to stay." She gazed at their reflection in the window glass. "'Tis' a humiliation I would not bear," she whispered. "Nor would I have you bear it for my sake."

Touched by her impassioned defense of him, Simon paused a moment to bring balance to the debate. "As kind as you are, Catherine, you must consider yourself, as well. You will be leaving your family, your friends—your entire life here, and although I understand that it is a voyage of but nine weeks, it may be a very long time, if ever, before we return. My brothers and sisters have all grown and made their way into the world. They no longer need me, but you need your family. As much as I am grateful for and adore your selflessness, this is not my decision to make. It is yours."

She clasped his hands in hers. "No, Simon, it is ours."

Her earnest eyes searched his. He relented. "Very well, but only if you speak your mind first."

Catherine paused a moment. "Then, I say…yes," she said, in a soft voice that betrayed the enormity of the moment.

"As do I."

They sat, stunned. It was that simple. *The decision was made.* "Then I shall go to the ticket office in the morning and purchase two tickets on the *Recovery.*" He took a deep breath. "We shall sail to America!" he cried out, unable to contain his excitement. He rose, pulling her into his arms. "You are an extraordinary woman," he whispered, as he kissed her tenderly. "You have changed my life in so many ways. I cannot begin to comprehend what will happen next."

Catherine pulled back from his grasp and tilted her head up to him, with a twinkle in her eyes. "If we wait much longer, you shall have to purchase three tickets."

CHAPTER FORTY-EIGHT

"AND IF THUS SMALL, THEN LADIES MAY WELL WEAR A
WORLD OF WORLDS, AS PENDANTS IN EACH EAR"
~ LADY MARGARET CAVENDISH

Blackwell Docks
London, England
Saturday, 16 April 1667

The blustery, spring air crackled with excitement at the Blackwell Docks. A stiff breeze blowing from the east sent loose handbills, showers of white hawthorn blossoms and scores of unpinned hats skittering across the wharves. Amid the smoky, burnt out warehouses and toppled brick administration buildings, reconstruction had at last begun. Soaring, skeletal racks of scaffolding, great piles of lumber and exhausted workers scurrying every which way added to the unending chaos. Through it all, the brisk trade in overseas migration had carried on.

Catherine stood on the dock and gripped the handle of her leather valise, waiting as Simon handed over the tickets to their small cabin on the captain's deck of the mighty sailing ship, *Recovery*. Her eyes traveled upwards in awe, for it was a truly magnificent galleon. Weighing over one hundred and forty tons, the dark, timbered ship sat high and silent in the water, waiting for the three cannon shots that would signal an imminent departure. At each end of the ship, 350 passengers stood at the roped-off gangplanks, their emotions running high. At precisely twelve o'clock, the first cannon shot thundered across the water, startling nearly everyone in line.

Exuberant shouts and cheers rang throughout the dockyard as the ropes were dropped, and the anxious passengers began to board. On the main deck, gaskets holding the sails to mast were unleashed by the seasoned jim-tars, and one by one, great sheets of canvas began to unfurl into a cerulean sky. Watching the sails billow and snap high above her, Catherine could hardly believe the day had at last come. As she had during these last three heady weeks of preparation, she fought once more to calm the uneasiness that crept into her thoughts, and steadied her jittery nerves with the promise they had made to stay for just one year. *She could not leave all she loved if it meant she would ne'er again see England.* Charles had sailed to the colonies and back, she reassured herself when troubled thoughts woke her in the night, and so could they. Until then, she avowed, she was determined to savor the adventure that lay so very far away.

Around her, the teeming docks were a delight to the senses. In the noisy, carnival-like atmosphere, bread sellers hawked their freshly baked, fragrant loaves to the departing passengers. Excited children flew kites on the blustery breezes as though they were on holiday. A few yards away, a fiddler played a jaunty tune while a monkey in a red cap danced for coins.

"Look lively, Miss!" cried a sailor carrying a crate of wine up to the captain's fo'sicle.

Catherine jumped back, and then ducked sideways to avoid two porters hauling a heavy trunk on their shoulders in last-minute preparations for the journey. She was unsure where to stand in the great crush of people.

"Mind yer step, Miss!" shouted one of the porters, jerking his chin toward something by her feet.

Catherine looked down to see a little boy about two years old sitting alone at her feet, playing with a stick. Alarmed, Catherine swung him up into her arms and began to search for his mother among the crowds disembarking from the nearby Dutch ship, *De Reusachtig.* The boy giggled, reaching this way and that for the tiny, white hawthorn petals that fluttered by.

"Jakob!" A young girl carrying a travel case shoved her way

through the confused swarm. "Jakob!" she screamed, racing toward Catherine and the boy. Scooping the child into her arms, the girl turned to Catherine with tears spilling from her eyes. "*Dank u, mevrouw*" she whispered. "Thank you, Miss. I am alone. He ran from me." She gestured to the crowds with a shaking hand. "I could not find him in the…the peoples," she said, in heavily accented English.

"He is a beautiful boy," smiled Catherine, captivated by his bright blue eyes and the whorls of blond curls that fell to his chin. She could not stop herself from reaching out to caress his chubby cheek. "He has such a sweet face." Catherine looked over to the Dutch galleon and the people still spilling down its ramps. "Have you just arrived?"

"*Ja, Missen.*" She shook her head and corrected herself. "Yes, Miss. My name is Geertje. I have come to be a seamstress," she said, balancing the boy on her hip. "I was told," she hesitated, "…by someone I loved that I must come to London. And so I have." Geertje looked to the vast destruction still left from the fire. "The peoples will need new clothes, *ja?*"

Catherine smiled softly, thinking of MaryPryde. She saw the same quiet determination in this girl. "Yes, Geertje, they very much will."

The boy began to kick and fuss, wanting to get down and run once more. Holding him tight, Geertje hoisted the travel case onto her shoulder and nodded. "I must leave. Thank you, Miss. Thank you for finding my Jakob."

"Goodbye, Geertje." Catherine watched the young mother and son disappear into the crowd, marveling at her courage.

"'Tis a girl, ye know."

Catherine jumped and looked down to see a misshapen, old woman dressed in rags, standing by her side. Startled by the woman's sudden appearance, Catherine tightened her hold on the valise and leaned down closer. "I beg your pardon?"

"Two a'penny, Miss," she whispered in a high, cracking

voice. "'Tis yer fortunes I'm seein', an' if ye'd like t' see 'em fer yerself, why it's two a'penny." The old woman grinned a toothless smile and held out a small, chipped teacup, nodding her encouragement.

Catherine was fascinated. "A girl? How did you…"

"Aye, Miss, an' me soothsayin's dead t' rights," she interrupted, drawing herself up proudly.

From behind, a single coin clunked dully into the porcelain cup. Catherine felt a hand grip her elbow.

"Thank you, ma'am," smiled Simon, drawing Catherine away from the crone.

The old woman sniffed her irritation at Simon, and then turned to a well-dressed gentleman making his way toward the *Recovery*. "'Tis a long voyage, ye'll be havin'…" she grinned, holding her cup high, hopeful of an easy mark. Pushed off by the man, she grudgingly pocketed her vessel and headed for the *De Reusachtig* in search of a few newly arrived and very gullible Dutch gudgeons.

"But, a girl—how could she have possibly known I am with child?" wondered Catherine aloud as Simon led her toward the first class passenger ramp. Her mind began to drift in tantalizing contemplations of a little red-haired daughter in her arms.

"You're young, you wear a wedding ring—t'was a safe enough prophesy," he laughed. "'Tis nearly time," he said, a catch in his calm voice betraying his great excitement.

A sharp whistle blew from the foredeck. Everyone looked up to the railing to see the captain dressed in his formal uniform. He surveyed the dock a moment, and then disappeared from sight. Above, the immense sails caught the wind and began to billow out, causing the ship to strain at the massive ropes holding it fast to the docks.

"Catherine!" waved Viola, standing with Charles, the mayor and Father Hardwicke. "Look who's come to see you off!" she cried out. Pippa and the ladies crowded around to bid them safe passage.

Amid the hugs and well wishes, Simon took Father Hardwicke aside for a private moment. "I cannot possibly thank you enough for everything you've done for me," said Simon, with a rasp in his throat. Simon clasped the old priest's hand in his own. "It would take a lifetime to repay my debt to you." In that moment, emotion overcame them both and the handshake became a hug that neither could bear let go of. "You have been more a father to me than my own," said Simon, clearing his throat to keep the tears at bay.

"I have never been more proud of a student," said Father Hardwicke. He paused a moment. "Or of a man," he whispered, choking back his own tears.

The mayor, uncomfortable with a serious moment, stepped to the two and clasped them both by the shoulders. "Aye lad, I suppose you'll be insistin' upon a dreary course of dull food," he rolled his eyes and then paused to retrieve a flacon from his cloak pocket, "and none of this," he grinned. With a twinkle in his eye, he removed the cork and offered it to the men. To his great surprise, Simon nodded, then took a generous sip, and offered it to the priest, who took a hefty swallow, himself. The mayor took the flacon back and raised it high. " Godspeed, Simon. Godspeed."

Catherine watched the three men share the moment, looking upon Simon with such pride. Viola quietly wrapped her arm around Catherine's waist and held her tight. "Will you be all right?" whispered Catherine.

"Cecil and I shall miss you terribly, my dear, but yes, we will be fine. However, if you are not back in one year, we shall have to sail to America ourselves!" she laughed.

The woman crowded around Catherine and Viola. "I shall miss you, terribly, myself," said Pippa, wiping a tear.

"As shall I," said Elizabeth, smiling through shining eyes. "Our Thursday gatherings won't be the same without you."

"Oh, but you have such an exciting journey ahead!" cried Aphra.

Catherine hugged each woman in turn, and then stopped, grasping Bathsua's hands. Catherine's eyes danced in anticipation. "I have spoken with both my aunt and Charles, and we have a proposal for you, dear Bathsua. Since Aunt Viola and the mayor are returning to the Abbey, and Charles will be lodging at the Inns of Court for the rest of his legal studies, Bealeton House will be empty for quite some time." Catherine took a deep breath, "We would like you to offer the use of Bealeton House for your girl's school until you can find permanent lodgings."

Bathsua looked from Catherine to Charles in disbelief. "I...I have no words for your kind offer," she paused, "but to say, thank you." She looked to them all. "Lady Hardwicke, Mayor Hardwicke, I am so grateful for your generosity."

"The house should not sit idle," said Viola, the catch in her brisk tone once more betraying her tenuous emotions. "I should think there would be room enough for ten girls."

The second cannon shot cracked over the bow. The thinning crowd on the dock jumped, and then fell silent at the enormity of the occasion. The time had come. Catherine hugged her brother," I shall miss you, Charles."

Though he would not dare admit it, Charles felt a bit at sea, himself. "I shall miss you, too," he said. "I wish you a safe journey. I...I love you, Catherine," he said, holding her tight. After a moment, Charles turned away to collect himself.

Catherine hugged the mayor and then her aunt. She could barely let go. "I will write when the baby comes," she whispered, tears filling her own eyes.

Still holding Catherine, Viola looked straight at Simon. "Are you certain she will be safe on the voyage?"

He nodded. "We have taken a small cabin on the upper deck. She will have plenty of time to rest, fresh air every day and we will eat with the captain most nights." He smiled. "I am sure you know, Lady Hardwicke, there are no certainties in childbirth," Simon reached for Catherine's hand, "but, I shall take very good care of her."

The final cannon shot sent ripples of excitement through the passengers crowding the rails.

Simon watched the smoke clear, then leaned down. "It is time," he said, gently easing Catherine toward the gangplank. Viola fought back tears as they all moved toward the step together, unwilling as she was to let go until the last second.

"Wait, wait!" cried a familiar voice over the din. "Wait!"

They looked back to see Gussie and Archie pushing their way through the crowd, bags in hand, and waving papers high in the air. "We're comin'!" They caught up to the stunned group, and stood, catching their breath. Gussie held out two tickets. "Ye did'na think I'd let ye have tha' wee bairn without me, did ye nae?" Gussie grinned, relishing the confused looks.

"I'm afraid I don't understand," said Catherine, knitting her brows. "How?"

Gussie looked to Archie, who laughed and nodded. "Go ahead, tell her."

"Well, ye see, lambkins, we had a good bit tucked away fera rainy day, an' with yer aunt and th' mayor returnin' to th' abbey, we thought ye'd be needin' us more, like as not." She put her hand on Archie's arm. "'Tis steerage, a'course, but yer not to worry, we'll be close enough by."

Catherine ran to her. "Oh, Gussie," she cried. "I'm so grateful," she said, through streaming tears.

A uniformed sailor leaned over the railing and clanged a bell. "Last call!" he shouted.

"It is time, Catherine," said Viola, linking her arm into Cecil's. "Carry on," she nodded, her brisk tone masking the soft emotion she tried to hide.

Catherine hugged her aunt and Charles once more, then, she and Simon stepped back. They took a deep breath and then, arm in arm, walked up the ramp. Gussie, Archie and the last few passengers boarded through the hatchway below. From the deck, Catherine waved down to the group on the dock as the ship creaked and strained against the pull of the ropes. The sailors pulled the ramps inside, and then secured the hatchways.

The captain appeared at the railing once more and gave one last whistle. "Cast off!" he cried. The sailors threw off the lines.

A strong wind caught the canvas square on and blew the flapping sails full. The wind whipped strands of hair across her face, as Catherine stood at the railing and breathed the intoxicating scent of fresh, salty air. Slowly, the galleon began to inch away from the dock. A shiver of excitement made her fingertips tingle. She looked out across the sparkling water toward a world far beyond anything she had ever known. *A new world.* A world where people lived their lives just as she had in England. It was nearly impossible to grasp. Worlds of people existed, yet they were unseen to her. India. China. America. Even the baby that was growing inside her. Each in their own world, yet she could neither see nor touch them. But she knew they were there. *How small the world was when one thought of it.*

She looked down to the dock. Charles, Viola, the mayor and her friends were still waving. She was leaving a world of everyone she loved, but she knew they would still be there. *They would always be there.* Simon slipped his arms around her waist and held her close as the ship began to move from the dock. He set a soft hand upon her stomach, a tender, protective gesture that reassured her anxious heart. Gathering speed, the galleon began to shift course and heave toward the open sea. Smiling up at him, she laid her head softly against his shoulder, and together, Catherine and Simon watched until the dock faded from sight.

AUTHOR'S NOTE

Having ended *The Boundary Stone* on August 27th, 1666, it was impossible in the sequel to not write about the Great Fire of London that broke out just five days later. The fire began on September 2nd at the Farynor bakery and, due to Lord Mayor Bloodworth's inaction (and yes, he really did say that), raged for five days, gutting nearly the entire medieval city. The fire consumed 13,200 houses, 87 parish churches, St. Pauls Cathedral and most city buildings. It is estimated to have destroyed the homes of 70,000 of the city's 80,000 citizens.

It seems impossible to contemplate that there were only seven small gates in the massive wall encircling London and although all those people were trying to storm the gates to escape, only six deaths were verified. The toll must have been much, much higher, however, as poor and middle-class deaths were not recorded at that time, and the heat of the fire most likely cremated many victims. A melted piece of pottery on display at the Museum of London found by archaeologists in Pudding Lane where the fire started, shows that the temperature reached 2,280°F. While nearly ⅞ths of the city inside the walls burned, the areas outside the wall, including St. Bartholomew's Hospital, Whitehall Palace and the West End, where this book was set, were left largely intact.

While researching material for *The Boundary Stone*, I came across a fascinating scientific experiment that had been performed in France, and I knew it would be a major plot point in *The Skeptical Physick*.

The 17th century was an amazing time for science and incredible advances in medicine were being discovered at a rapid pace. The Scientific Revolution that was taking place in Europe was well underway and marked the emergence of modern science over superstition and speculation. The Royal

Society of London for Improving Natural Knowledge (The Royal Society), had just been founded in 1660 and had been granted a royal charter by King Charles II.

In 1667, a French physician, Jean-Baptiste Denys, was experimenting with blood transfusion, and while the actual experiment took place several months after it occurs in *The Skeptical Physick*, some of the key details served as the basis for the novel. In actuality, Denys performed two transfusions using the blood of a sheep on a mentally ill patient in hopes of making him more docile. When the patient survived the first two attempts, Denys tried once more. After the third attempt, the patient died, and Denys was tried for murder—however, it turned out, according to medical historian Holly Tucker, that the patient died of arsenic poisoning administered by competing physicians who were jealous of the notoriety Denys had achieved. Denys was later acquitted. What a great twist, and one I had to use for the book!

King Charles II (1630-1685) was one of the most popular and beloved kings of England, and a complete breath of fresh air after the strict, humorless, dictatorial Oliver Cromwell. There were those, like Lord Clarendon, who despised his mistress, the Countess of Castlemaine, and the king's hedonistic ways (he acknowledged at least twelve illegitimate children by various mistresses), however, he mitigated his failings with his lively sense of fun and curiosity, earning himself the title of "The Merry Monarch." What he went through to regain the throne is a story not to be believed and his interest in science was just as fascinating as the other aspects of his life. His personal efforts, along with his brother James, in fighting the fire, as well as his foresight in rebuilding London afterward forever endeared him his subjects.

I was also fascinated by Lady Elizabeth Wilbraham (1632-1705), and knew I had to include her in the book, as well. She was a beautiful, intelligent member of the English aristocracy, who became the first female architect, ever. Her husband, who agreed to extend their honeymoon to six years so that she could study architecture in Italy, Germany and the Netherlands, wholeheartedly supported her in her architectural pursuits. As many as 400 buildings, including 12 family homes are attributed to her, and because of the inclusion of distinctive and unusual design details, historian John Millar proposes that she may also have been the designer of 18 London churches (attributed to Christopher Wren), including St. Paul's Cathedral. Wren came late to architecture, and because of a close association, Millar suggests Lady Wilbraham as his most likely architectural tutor. During the 17th century, it was all but impossible for a woman to pursue a profession and Lady Wilbraham is said to have used male executant architects to supervise construction (and take credit) in her place. The other women, Aphra Behn and Bathsua Makin were accomplished in their own rights, and their lives are equally impressive.

It is easy to think of history as full of nameless, faceless ancestors who trudged through life, but human nature is human nature no matter the century, and I hope I brought to life some of the fictional and real people, especially the women, who laughed, cried, created, dreamed and achieved the same way we do now.

If you enjoyed *The Skeptical Physick*, I'd love to hear from you! Please feel free to contact me for book clubs or speaking engagements at gailaveryhalverson@gmail.com and follow @gailaveryhalverson (IG) or gailaveryhalverson (FB). Kind reviews on Amazon and Goodreads of *The Boundary Stone* and *The Skeptical Physick* are always very appreciated.